One on One
WITH
Tony Little

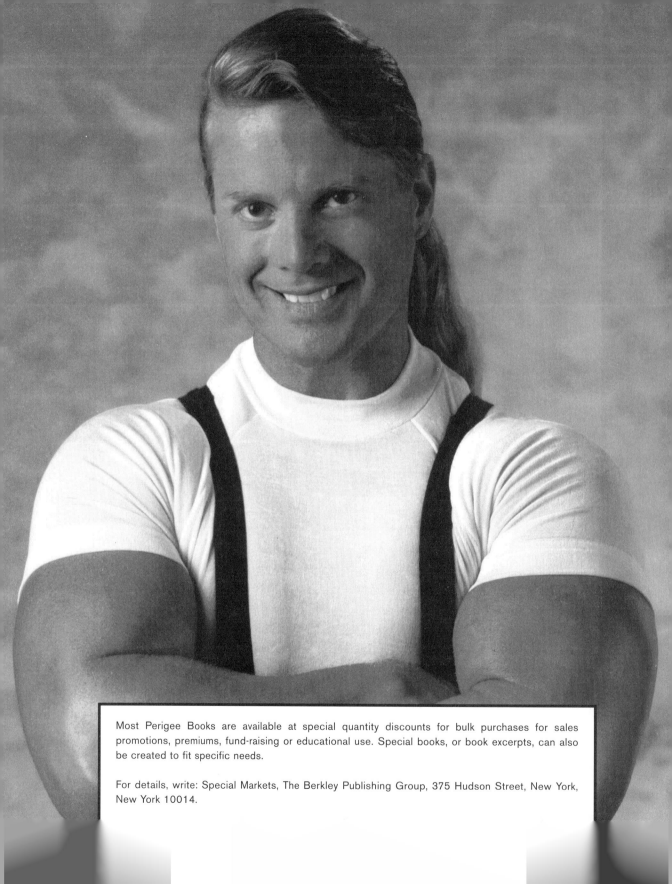

One on One

WITH

Tony Little

A Complete 28-Day
Body Sculpting and
Weight Loss
Program

by

Tony Little

America's Personal Trainer™

PERIGEE BOOKS
NEW YORK

A Perigee Book
Published by The Berkley Publishing Group
A division of Penguin Group (USA) Inc.
375 Hudson Street
New York, New York 10014

Copyright © 2003 by Health International Corporation
Cover design by Wendy Bass
Cover photo by Robert Rieff
Text design by Pauline Neuwirth

First Perigee edition: December 2003

ISBN: 0-399-52921-7

Visit our website at www.penguin.com

Library of Congress Cataloging-in-Publication Data

One-on-one with Tony Little: a complete 28-day body sculpting and weight loss
    program / Tony Little.—1st ed.
        p. cm.
    "A Perigee book."
    Includes index.
    ISBN 0-399-52921-7
    1. Bodybuilding—Handbooks, manuals, etc. 2. Weight loss—
Handbooks, manuals, etc. I. Title.

GV546.5.L55 2003
613. 7'1—dc21
                                                        2003048654

Printed in the United States of America

10   9   8   7   6   5   4   3   2   1

Acknowledgments

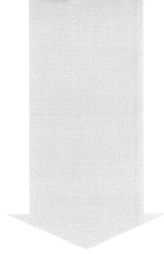

THIS LIST IS in random order. There is no way to prioritize my gratitude to the many people in my life who have helped me become the person I am today.

I am grateful to all the people who believed in me and supported me through the good and the bad times—you know who you are! The best thank you I can give is to call you my friends.

This same thankfulness extends to all the people who have put their trust in me, followed my programs and purchased my products. The Wall of Fame in this book is a tribute to many of them. Their success stories, letters, calls, and e-mails have lifted my spirit through the years.

I can't let this book go to print without mentioning my daughter, Tara, and son, Trent, who will always be my most cherished assets. They both have provided me, and continue to provide me, the inspiration to keep going forward, no matter what happens to me in life.

To my brother and sisters, thank you for always being there for me.

Kim: through good times and bad, you have helped me get to where I am today. I am forever grateful.

Sue, Hank, and John: I cannot imagine life without you guys around. Thank you for all you have done for me through the years.

This book would not exist without the help of Laura Dayton, who takes my ideas and thoughts and helps put them into words that would make an English teacher proud. God knows, my English teacher was not proud very often! Laura's contributions have been integral. This is a special thanks to her at this time, as I know she's weathering a rough time in her own life but still makes the time for me.

I would also like to thank Lifestyle Family Fitness Center in Seminole, Florida, for the opportunity to shoot some of the exercise photos at their awesome facility. Also, John and Tina Clifford and George Zickl for the great photos.

If I didn't mention my incredible office staff, not only would I find my chair being pulled out from under me and my protein shakes served warm but also it would be a terrible injustice. To those who have gone before and who will come in the future, thank you. I've been blessed to always have such helpful and loyal staff.

To Ray Manzella, my manager, for his help in putting the pieces of this together, and for being there for me through the years.

To Sheila and the rest of the staff at Perigee, thank you for giving me this opportunity to share a practical guide to lifestyle changes that will impact so many people in so many great ways.

And of course, a big thank you to all the people I've forgotten to mention!

I started by saying this list was random, but it's not. First, last, and always is my thankfulness to God for giving me hope and determination, and now at an older age, wisdom.

Contents

Wall of Fame

Here are some of the people who followed a

Tony Little program to realize their dreams.

Let them be an inspiration to you for the next

28 days. They inspire me as well!

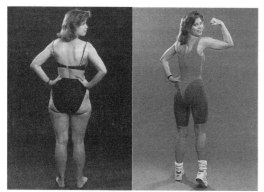

Sherry from FL lost 26 inches

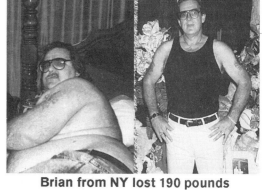

Brian from NY lost 190 pounds

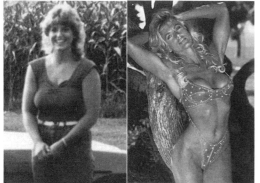

Jena from IN lost 60 pounds

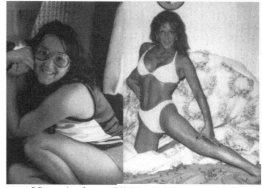

Maggie from NY lost 30 pounds

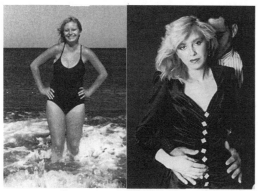

Laurie from Canada lost 35 pounds

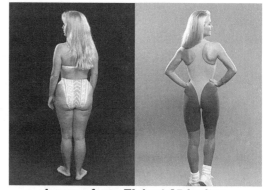

Jeanne from FL lost 35 inches

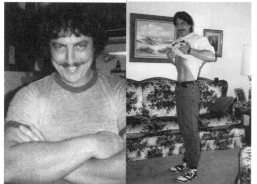

Mike from IN lost 70 pounds

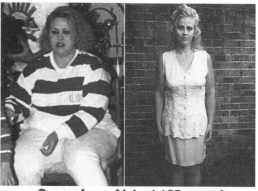

Susan from AL lost 125 pounds

WALL OF SUCCESS

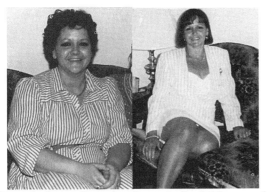

Brenda from Ontario, Canada lost 51 pounds

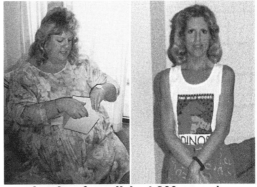

LeeAnn from IL lost 200 pounds

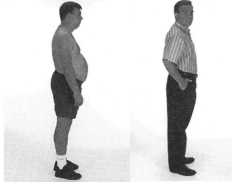

Don from FL lost 21.5 inches

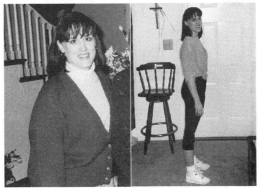

Connie from IN went from a size 16 to 10

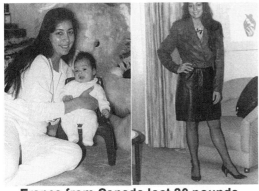

Franca from Canada lost 30 pounds

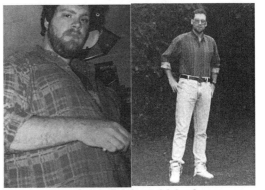

Dan from PA lost 20 inches

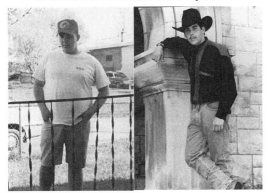

Daniel from OH lost 110 pounds

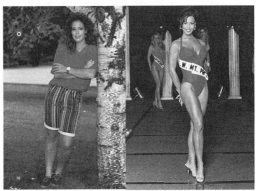

Heather from CA lost 50 pounds

INTRODUCTION
Why You Need
This Book

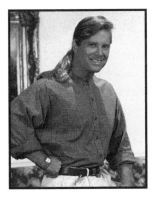

AS A PERSONAL trainer I've seen nearly every book on fitness, every book on weight loss, and every book on getting in shape. I'm still stunned by the massive amount of information authors try to supply without ever providing the reader with a simple, one-on-one *let's-learn-as-we-do* strategy!

The truth is, the simplest and most effective way to get real results in weight loss and body sculpting is to do it daily, learn a little daily, and see results daily. This book gives you the same type of personal training program that I would use if you were paying me hundreds of dollars per session!

One-on-One with Tony Little is written as if I were with you in person every day. No guesswork. Just you and me—and my professional advice on what to eat, exercises to do, and motivation that will encourage you to finally experience the *power* of *one-on-one* personal training. We will work together to help you achieve the results you've wanted for so long.

I'm fortunate to have helped millions of people worldwide to change their minds and change their bodies through personal training videos and DVDs. You'll be inspired and motivated by many of the true success stories included in this book. You'll learn in a very simple, practical manner how to enjoy more weight loss and greater rewards than with any other book or program you've used in the past—guaranteed!

Conceive, believe, and achieve!

There's always a way!

READY, GET SET, GO!

This book will take you step by step through a 28-day program. Each day is spelled out for you and broken into four sections: Brain Power, Eating Right, Workouts, and Health Smarts.

BRAIN POWER

Brain Power will give you the encouragement, motivation, and mental tips that will help you to achieve that positive mind-set necessary to reach your goals quickly. Set time aside each day, preferably in the morning, to review the day's Brain Power—even if it means you have to get up a few minutes early! Doing this will help you to reflect on your goals and your progress to start your day in the right frame of mind.

EATING RIGHT

Eating Right will provide you with the suggested meal plans for the day. Each meal is formulated to keep you on the 40-40-20 way of eating—that is, 40% protein, 40% carbohydrates, and 20% fat. We will discuss this in detail later, but in a nutshell, here is how it works. Use your fist as a portion guideline. At each meal, have a fist-sized portion of protein and a fist-sized portion of carbohydrates, chosen from the low-glycemic list of carbohydrates in this book. There is no need for a portion of fat because the fat comes naturally with the protein and carbohydrates! Listen to your body! Don't overeat. Stop when you feel satisfied, not when you feel like you have to unbutton your pants and lay down. And remember, we want to stay away from the diet mentality.

WORKOUTS

Exercise is so important to your body, physically and mentally. I will give you suggestions on cardiovascular exercise to burn those calories, and resistance exercise to increase your muscle tone, improve your body's shape, and speed up your metabolism for 24-hour calorie burning. Both are important to you for achieving your goals.

HEALTH SMARTS

I've included lots of "no B.S." information that will be important for getting you on the road to better health and fitness for life. I have also dispelled myths about exercise and eating to giving you the facts on how your body works. Health Smarts will give you the knowledge you need to achieve your goals. Knowledge is power and this book is packed with power—the power to change your body and mind, now!

IT'S EASY AND EFFECTIVE

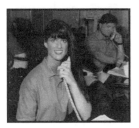

There is nothing complicated about this program, and I'm there for you every step of the way—as are my personal trainers who are available to you daily at our toll-free number: 1-800-780-6744.

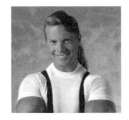

ASK YOUR PERSONAL TRAINER™

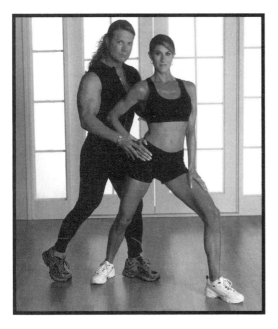

You may perform this program from the comfort of your own living room or at your local health club. Each day's instructions are at your fingertips with no tedious reading or study. It's just you and me—ONE ON ONE.

For the home workout you will need some light dumbbells or elastic exercise bands. Pairs of three-, five-, and eight-pound dumbbells are good starting choices for women. Ten- and 12-pound dumbbells are ideal for men. Elastic bands, which are available at any sporting goods store, come with complete instructions for varying the resistance. The moves are the same for both. You will also need a small bench or armless chair.

I will also show you how to do some of these exercises at the gym. Be sure not to overwork a body part by doing both versions of the exercise.

IT'S NOW OR NEVER!

For the next 28 days every day is a *now-or-never* day! Take this book and its daily messages to bed with you every night. Wake up each day with a new outlook that brings energy and confidence into your life!

Come on! Let's get started!

Tony Little

One on One
WITH
Tony Little

BEFORE YOU BEGIN

1

Let's synchronize our lives so we start out together!

I'd like you to begin the program on a Monday. This will allow us to factor in those nine-to-five weekday schedules that many of us live by and the rest of us schedule around. This also lets you have more freedom for the weekends.

Monday is significant because it represents a new beginning.

KITCHEN CLEANOUT— SO YOU CAN LEAN OUT!

Before we start I'd like you to pick a day—preferably during the weekend before you begin the program—to put your *now-or-never* attitude on. Let's do some very important cleaning of your kitchen cupboards and fridge!

Yep. You heard me right. Not only is this a very important step, it may be the most important step of the entire program!

I want you to clean out the "bad-body" foods and bad habits from your kitchen. That's right. You're going to give away or throw away the things that are preventing you from losing weight and reaching for greater shape-up goals!

Remove everything from your cupboards and fridge, then read the label on each item to ascertain whether it has any nutritional value or if it's just empty calories. Keep only premium fuels; your body is an ultimate driving machine and you need to give it the best fuel you can find. Here's a list to help you identify the good, the bad, and the middle of the road.

BAD-BODY FOODS

PROTEINS

- Fatty beef/pork/veal products
- Breaded meats (breaded chicken, chicken parmesan, country fried steak)
- Real cream
- Whole milk
- Whole cheese and cheese products

FATS

- Anything—except oils—that derives more than 95% of its calories from fat
- Anything—including oils—that derives the majority of its fat from saturated fat
- Real mayonnaise
- Margarine

CARBOHYDRATES

- Foods that list maltodextrin and/or partially hydrogenated fats (trans fat) within the first four ingredients on the label

- High-fructose fruit juices or anything that's not 100% fruit juice
- Any candies, cookies, or desserts that are not packaged in small bite-sized portions and are high in carbohydrates and fat
- Waffle/pancake mix
- Ice cream
- Frozen yogurt bars
- Sugary breakfast cereals (read the labels)
- Donuts and other pastries
- Canned fruits in heavy syrup

OTHER FOODS TO TOSS OUT

- Most prepared meal "helpers" ("just add the meat")
- Foods with more than 600 grams of sodium a serving
- Rice cakes (yes, believe it or not!)
- Non-diet soft drinks

GOOD-BODY FOODS

PROTEINS

- Lean meats (chicken and turkey without skin, lean beef, fish)
- Milk, nonfat or 2%
- Tofu
- Egg substitutes or eggs, poached, boiled, or Pam-fried
- Reduced-calorie frozen dinners (just watch sodium content)
- Low-sodium soups
- Low-carbohydrate, high-protein meal replacement bars, drinks, and shakes
- Low-fat cottage cheese
- Low-fat cream cheese
- Low-fat yogurt, preferably plain
- Peanut butter

FATS

- Pam spray
- Olive oil
- Butter (this is not permission to eat all the butter you want!)
- Molly McButter Sprinkles
- Smart Balance margarine brands

- Other butter substitutes
- Just 2 Good or other reduced-fat mayonnaise/salad dressings

CARBOHYDRATES

- Fresh fruits, especially winter melons and all berries
- Fresh vegetables, especially those that can be eaten raw, such as carrots, celery, broccoli, and tomatoes
- Canned or frozen fruits and vegetables, not packed in salt or sugar
- Pastas (in moderation)
- Sourdough, rye, pumpernickel, or whole-grain breads
- Oatmeal and all-bran cereals
- Beans, lentils, and bulgur
- Sweet potatoes
- Small baked potatoes or half a big potato

OTHER KEEPERS

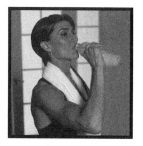

- Any foods that contain a 40-40-20 or 50-30-20 balance of protein, carbohydrates, and fat (see Day 7)
- All types of low-sodium bottled waters (distilled water is great for the first 28 days! Water, water, water and plenty of it!)
- A good multiple vitamin/mineral supplement
- Meal replacement bars and drinks

A note about bars and shakes: Just because they are in a health food store, or in the health food aisle at the grocery store, does not necessarily mean they are healthy. Look for bars or shakes that have a minimum protein gram count of 15, and look for bars or shakes that have zero sugar carbohydrates. There is a fairly new concept in the low-carbohydrate category of foods called net carbohydrates. The manufacturer will take the total carbohydrates, and subtract the fiber, and any other carbohydrates that have little to no effect on your blood sugar, and the number they come up with from there is the net carbs. Look for bars or shakes that have less than four net carbohydrates.

If the rest of your household doesn't want to participate in the program, then set aside a special area for "your" food, then vow to only eat from that selection of food. If you stock your shelves with only healthy choices, the battle is nearly won.

For more good-body choices, check out the following on low-glycemic carbohydrates chart.

Low-Glycemic Carbohydrates Chart

What is the Glycemic Index?

Simply put, the Glycemic Index of a food measures how it will affect the glucose levels in your blood (your blood sugar). The index number is obtained through testing, by using a standard food (normally glucose) and then comparing the blood glucose effect of other foods to the standard. The higher the number, the more it affects your blood-sugar levels. Carbohydrates stimulate increases in blood sugar, and some of them are not good for low-carbohydrate diets.

Very Low, Very Good, Eat All You Want!

Yogurt, low fat, artificially sweetened	20	Kidney beans	42
Soybeans	25	Black beans	43
Rice bran	27	Apricots, dried	44
Cherries	32	Milk, skim	46
Fructose	32	Lima beans, baby, frozen	46
Peas, dried	32	Fettuccine	46
Barley, pearl	36	Chickpeas (garbanzo beans)	47
Grapefruit	36	Rye	48

Low, Good, and Eat Freely

Pears, fresh	53	Macaroni	64
Spaghetti, whole meal	53	Linguine	65
Apples	54	Lactose	65
Haricot/navy beans	54	Grapes	66
Plums	55	Pineapple juice	66
Pinto beans	55	Bulgur	68
Kellogg's All-Bran Fruit 'n Oats	55	Rice, parboiled	68
Apple juice	58	Peas, green	68
Black-eyed peas	59	Grapefruit juice	69
All-Bran	60	Pumpernickel	71
Peaches, fresh	60	Ice cream, low fat	71
Oranges	63	Orange juice	74

continued

Borderline High, Still Okay to Eat

Special K	77	Popcorn	79
Bananas	77	Apricots, fresh	82
Sweet potatoes	77	Honey	83
Oat Bran	78	Rice, white	83
Buckwheat	78	Split pea soup	86
Sweet corn	78	Porridge (oatmeal)	87
Rice, brown	79	Ice cream	87

Too High, Avoid These

Raisins	91	Watermelon	103
Beets	91	Swede (rutabaga)	103
Sucrose (table sugar)	92	Cheerios	106
Couscous	93	French fries	107
Pineapple	94	Donuts	108
Grape Nuts	96	Waffles	109
Stoned Wheat Thins	96	Total brand cereal	109
Cornmeal	98	Broad beans (fava beans)	113
Wheat bread, whole-meal flour	99	Pretzels	116
Shredded Wheat	99	Rice Krispies	117
Melba toast	100	Cornflakes	119
Cream of Wheat	100	Potatoes, baked	121
Millet	101	Glucose	137
Carrots	101	Parsnips	139
Wheat bread, white	101	Glucose tablets	146
Bagel, white	103	Maltose	150

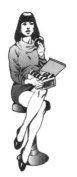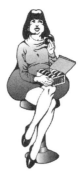

Eat a donut, look like a donut.
Illustration by Matt Gouig

The Way You Cook Also Counts!

It's not just the food you eat, but the way you prepare it. Here is a simple list of the good, and the bad that makes the ugly.

Good Cooking
Broiling
Baking
Grilling
Stir-frying (lite oil)
Steaming (veggies)
Boiling (meats)
Pressure cooking

Bad Cooking
Frying
Deep frying
Battering any food
Open-fire grilling

CURRENT BODY MEASUREMENTS

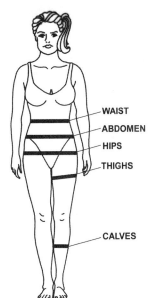

Now that you've got your kitchen under control it's time to move on to the real deal. Each day I'll be filling you in on what to focus on, what to eat, and how to exercise. At the end of each day is a space for you to keep track of your progress—you will be amazed at what you can do. Taking your measurements is an excellent way to keep track of your changing shape as you get fit.

For starters, take your baseline measurements. Your measurements (not your bathroom scale) will be the best assessment of your progress. When you burn fat and increase your muscle mass you may weigh a bit more even though your body is getting tighter and smaller. You can keep track of them on this page or a separate sheet by date.

Measure yourself on Day 1, first thing in the morning in the spots indicated in the illustration. It is important to measure yourself in the right spots, and consistently, to really gauge your results. Here is how you take seven different body measurements. Remember to keep your muscles relaxed while you're measuring.

1. CHEST: Measure all the way around your bust and back right at your nipple line. Don't squish yourself, and make sure the tape measure is not lower in the back.
2. UPPER ARMS: Measure wherever they are biggest above your elbows
3. WAIST: Measure wherever it is the smallest. If you have "no waist" go around yourself right at the navel line.
4. ABDOMEN: Measure midway between the very biggest part of your hips and your waist.
5. HIPS: Measure at the very biggest part, even if that is so low that you are almost on the top of your thighs.
6. THIGHS: Measure wherever they are the biggest.
7. CALVES: Measure wherever they are the biggest.

Don't re-measure every day! If you can wait until the 28th day, that would be best. It may seem discouraging to see your measurements when you start a fitness plan, but once you begin to see results, the feeling of accomplishment makes it all worth it. Get your tape measure and start measuring!

	START	DAY 28
Chest		
Arms		
Waist		
Abdomen		
Hips		
Thighs		
Calves		
Dress Size		
Pant Size		
Weight		

Oh, and one more thing: pick out a pair of pants or shorts, a business suit, or some other article of clothing that does not fit you. However, maybe not that pair of size 4 jeans you wore in high school! Set a realistic goal. And instead of the scale, use that article of clothing to assess your progress through the next four weeks!

WEEK 1:
Starting Out

2

Our 28-day program has a learning curve, so there's a lot of information at the beginning and things get easier as each day goes by. You might be wondering why I chose 28 days, instead of 30 or 31 as in most calendar months. The answer is simple: it only takes four weeks to make a habit—you have just 28 days until you make healthy living your lifestyle!

DAY 1

BRAIN POWER

Today is the day you start to change your life for the better. This, and every day for the next 28 days, is your *now-or-never* day.

Today is the single most important day to change your mind, your body and your future.

The only way to fail on this system is to quit, and you are not a quitter! You're a winner! Life is short and death is way too long, so seize the moment, believe in yourself and *you will win*! I need you to trust me on this one; 28 days is not a long time, and you can do anything for 28 days! Once we get there, you will feel so good you won't want to stop. Think positive; don't let anyone or anything bring you down. These next 28 days are all about you! Focus all your energy on making YOU the person you have longed to be.

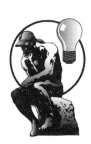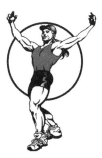

Think great, look great!
Illustration by Matt Gouig

EATING RIGHT

Make no mistake, you are absolutely what you eat!

I am not putting you on a diet in the usual sense; I am giving you a sensible nutrition plan. Each day I will outline your meals and include alternatives. I'll also provide nutritional tips to help you make better food choices. We've cleaned out your cabinets and fridge to make your food choices easier; when there are only healthy choices, eating well is a cinch! I'm also giving you options of what to eat if you are on the go and what to eat if you can have the time to fix a meal.

I want you to write down in a book what you eat every day. This book will be like a journal. Carry it with you everywhere you go to make it easier to chart your progress. Got it? Be sure to write down everything you eat today, all your exercise, and what you think about!

**You are what you eat.
You are what you do.
You are what you think.
Keep track of it!**

BREAKFAST

Eat breakfast. Got that? Don't forget it!

Breakfast is your fuel for the start of your day. If you skip breakfast, your tank is on empty. This is a fact, Jack! You will have *no* energy, and no energy eventually makes you fat. Your choice of food for breakfast will also dramatically affect the way you feel at the start of the day. Look for breakfast items that are high in protein and low in sugars.

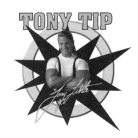

Eat breakfast after your workout, not before. It's okay to have a piece of fruit before a workout. And if you want something to warm you up and energize your workout, a cup of coffee or tea is ideal—just skip or go real easy on the cream and if you haven't already, try and switch to a sugar substitute.

Breakfast on the go: If you are a person on the go, or someone who doesn't usually eat breakfast, reach for a high-protein, low-carbohydrate meal replacement smoothie or bar. Remember to drink at least one big glass of water with breakfast, and don't forget to take a multiple vitamin/mineral supplement. If you are not used to taking a supplement at breakfast, make sure you take it with food, as it can upset your stomach!

Sit-down breakfast: For your protein, have three eggs (or egg substitute), poached, fried with Pam spray, or scrambled. For your carbohydrate, have one slice of sourdough or rye bread with I Can't Believe It's Not Butter spray or a spread that does not contain trans fat (also known as partially hydrogenated oil). You can have one cup of coffee or tea, black or with a low-fat cream substitute and sugar substitute, if necessary. You may also have a six-ounce glass of orange juice, or apple juice, or a piece of fruit. Try to eat the fruit and carbohydrates before the protein, if possible. Don't forget a daily multiple vitamin/mineral supplement every morning!

Now get to work and have a killer day! You are a go-getter and a winner!

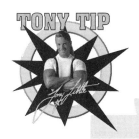

Try drinking distilled water over the next 28 days. Drink eight to preferably 16 ounces with every meal. It helps to purge the system of sodium so you'll have less bloat and a nicer body to tote!

LUNCH

Lunch on the go: Grab that high-protein, low-carbohydrate meal replacement smoothie or bar. Be sure to drink plenty of water with lunch and throughout the day!

Restrict your on-the-go meal replacement bars to no more than two a day. You may choose ready-to-drink smoothies and shakes and keep a stockpile in your fridge. Or, you may mix your own with ice, water, or nonfat milk and a high-protein, low-carbohydrate powder with frozen strawberries.

Sit-down lunch: Add a small amount of low-fat mayonnaise or salad dressing to a six- or eight-ounce can of water-packed tuna, mix with peas and/or chopped celery, and spread onto two slices of whole grain, sourdough, rye, or pumpernickel bread for a high-protein, low-carbohydrate lunch. Hint: add a little mustard or pickle relish to moisten your tuna salad.

If you don't like tuna, try a chicken breast—grilled, baked or broiled without the skin—on two slices of bread with lettuce, tomato, and mayonnaise. Turkey is also okay as long as it's breast meat.

Have an apple or orange for dessert. Drink at least eight ounces of water.

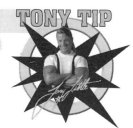

TONY TIP

Feeling hungry? Remember, you are what you eat. If you need a snack, keep it healthy and make it fresh fruit, veggies, or half a protein bar or shake.

SUPPER

Supper on the go: Drink a high-protein, low-carbohydrate smoothie or shake, or eat one high-protein, low-carbohydrate meal replacement bar. Remember, never exceed two meal replacement bars per day and that you need to have at least one sit-down meal a day!

Be sure to drink eight ounces or more of water with your meal replacement!

Sit-down supper: Grill or broil a two- to three-ounce cube steak patty (you may substitute tuna steak, salmon, chicken breast, or turkey). Add a fist-size portion of green beans, lima beans, spinach, or salad with oil and vinegar, fat-free Italian dressing, or balsamic vinegar. Have a sweet or baked potato with butter substitute or trans-fat-free spread (read the label). Try a bit of A-1 sauce on your potato—it tastes great! Don't go overboard on the A-1; there is lots of hidden sugar in there! Again, drink plenty of water. Water helps you lose body fat and it is great for your skin. A hydrated body is a happy body.

WORKOUT

CARDIOVASCULAR EXERCISE

Today we begin to work on our cardiovascular endurance and our core body strength area: our abs, back, and legs.

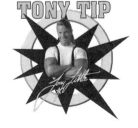

It is best to do cardio work in the morning because it is the single-best time of the day to charge up your metabolism and burn fat. Cardio on a nearly empty stomach may even give you an extra fat burn.

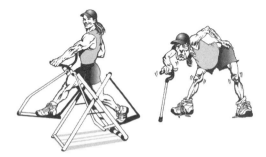

If you don't use it, you lose it!
Illustration by Matt Gouig

Begin with 12 minutes of continuous lower body movement. There is no stopping until 12 minutes are achieved so set your watch!

Choices of exercises include marching around your living room, stationary cycling, walking outside, walking on a treadmill, gliding on the Gazelle Glider, a or using the elliptical machine. Put on your headphones, crank up some music, and get started! Remember: keep movements fluid, energized, and brisk—not fast, just comfortable. Always choose low-impact cardio (no jolting, pounding or jarring the knees and ankles).

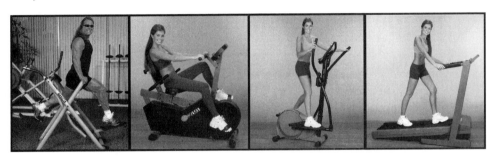

Don't forget to write down your cardio exercise on your training log!

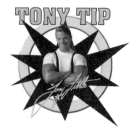

If you suffer from back pain, do not use step machines or walk on inclines! When lifting any object off the floor, use your legs! This protects your back.

RESISTANCE EXERCISE

If you're a person with a busy schedule, it is best to get this done right after your cardio in the morning. You'll have fewer chances to concoct excuses, and you'll feel the energy and enjoy the accomplishment all day long.

Resistance exercise will also increase your lean muscle mass, which adds shape to your body, burns calories even while you're not exercising, and helps restore growth hormones to keep you looking and feeling young!

HAND WEIGHTS

At the beginning of your excercise program, use no weights, and concentrate of proper technique and form. Learn your excercises well, using the *squeeze* methods. This should take two to four workouts. Once you are comfortable with technique, you can begin to use hand weights to enhance your workout. Weights can be purchased at your local sporting goods store, or even at your local retailer, such as Target, Wal-Mart, or K-Mart.

Beginners should use 3- to 5-pound weights, depending on the muscle being worked and the strength of the muscle. Those at the intermediate level (semiathletic or experienced excerciser) should begin by using 5- to 10-pound weights. If you are at the advanced level, you can start with 10- to 15-pound weights, depending on the muscle being worked and the strength of the muscle.

Your last two to three repetions in a set should be difficult. If they are not, move up to the next level with your weights.

Note: Some men or women may find these weights too light at 15 repetitions. If so, go up in weight resistance. Never sacrifice form for higher weights.

WEIGHTS AT THE GYM

For gym workouts, find a weight that is most comfortable to perform all the repetions of an exercise, using the *squeeze* technique. Remeber that form is more important than higher weight. The 12th-15th repetions should be difficult to perform. if they are not difficult bump up the weight.

> # Exercise is a fountain of youth.
> # Bathe in it every day!

Technique is the key. You must work your mind *and* muscles, always squeezing as many muscle groups as possible with each movement. All exercises may be performed in the home or at a health club! Think *squeeze* when you perform any exercise in order to work the muscle most effectively.

Today, perform only one set of each exercise.

1. Ab crunches (midsection):

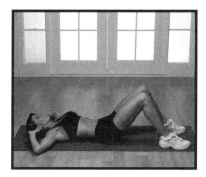 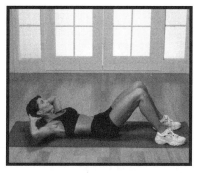

When you crunch, think *squeeze!* Lie on your back with your knees bent as shown. Press your whole back to the floor, leaving no space between you and the floor! Keep your chin up. Keep your eyes to the ceiling. Keep your neck in a neutral position. Place your hands lightly against your head. Do not use your hands to pull your head forward. Roll your shoulders forward, bringing your head toward your knees (or better, your chin up towards the ceiling). Keep your lower back on the floor, feet planted solidly.

Throughout this exercise, keep the muscles of your abs and buttocks tense. At the peak of the crunch, exhale and *squeeze* even harder. Use 100% of your concentration to keep your body as tense as possible and to keep these movements slow and precise. *Think about those abs!*

SET ONE: 10-15 repetitions

2. Reverse crunch (midsection):

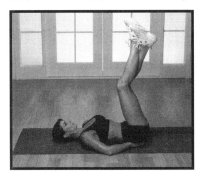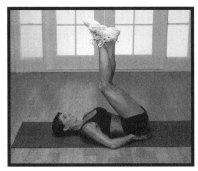

This exercise works the lower portion of the abs. Lie with your hands under your lower back (as shown). Think *squeeze* and send a mental message to make all the muscles of your torso tense. With your legs together, knees slightly bent, slowly rock your knees up toward your shoulders, being careful not to allow your lower back to leave the mat. No jerky motions! Go for a controlled lift, and lift your heels closer to the ceiling.

Think technique!

SET ONE: 10-15 repetitions

3. Lying back extension (lower back):

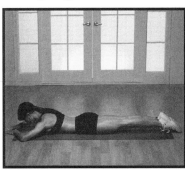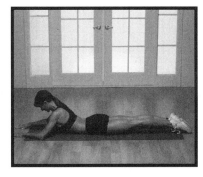

Always work your lower back when you work your abs. Lie face down on a mat or towel on the floor. Place your arms in front of you (as shown). Keeping your legs straight, push your upper torso up until you feel your glutes (that is your buttocks!) contract. Really *squeeze* at this point and hold for one second before repeating.

SET ONE: 10-15 repetitions

4. One-half squats (front and back of upper legs):

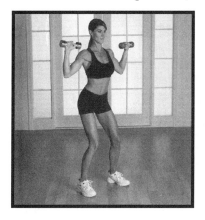 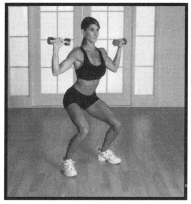

Strong legs support core strength, and the squat is the king of the leg exercises. We'll begin with a one-half squat. Use your own body weight or light, 5- to 15-pound dumbbells. With feet shoulder-width apart, stand as shown. Slowly squat down as though you were about to sit in a chair. Go only halfway down (as shown). Don't let your knees go out past your toes. Stand sideways in front of a mirror to be sure there is no unnecessary strain on your knees. Then, push with your legs and glutes back up to a standing position and squeeze. I mean *squeeze!* Squeeze all the way up your legs, to your glutes. Get the maximum results, don't settle for less.

Start with no weights. Use just your bodyweight, and reach your hands out or up for balance. Once you can do the reps without working too hard, add light 5- to 15-pound dumbbells. If you do not have any dumbbells, soup cans work just as well!

SET ONE: 10-15 repetitions

Told you you could do it! The more you believe in yourself—and the more you perform these exercises—the stronger you get physically and mentally each and every day. I promise you, your accomplishments in this program will bring joy and meaning into your life as never before!

If you need a snack before bed, have half a cantaloupe, an orange, apple, or half a protein bar. It is important to eat your last meal or snack of the day at least two to three hours before bed! If you get hungry, drink water.

It's not only what you eat but when you eat that counts!

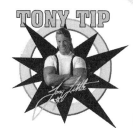

TONY TIP

YOU ARE WHAT YOU KNOW! SO KNOW *THAT PROTEIN IS KING*

As a former competitive bodybuilder, I learned very early the importance of protein. Protein feeds our muscles. It contains only four calories per gram, and unless consumed in huge excess, is stored as healthy, strong muscle, not jiggly, lazy fat.

It also slows down the absorption of other nutrients, keeping our insulin levels steady. This is so important today when the United States is experiencing an epidemic of diabetes!

Maintaining a healthy level of muscle mass though exercise and protein intake is necessary for maintaining a healthy bodyweight. Because muscles work, which means they expend energy (even at rest), one pound of muscle burns on average 30 to 50 calories a day. That means ten pounds of lean muscle burns an extra 300 to 500 calories a day, while not exercising. A pound of fat burns zero!

Balance, Balance, Balance

Like fat and sugar, protein comes in two varieties. For protein, the varieties are complete and incomplete. The protein from animals and animal byproducts is complete, meaning it contains all the essential amino acids necessary for the body to use it. That is one of the reasons why milk- and egg-protein supplements are so popular—they supply complete proteins to help build and restore your body's muscle tissue.

If you don't eat dairy, you need to be more creative. Eating compatible food sources can turn incomplete proteins into complete. Humans intuitively have known this fact for centuries.

Bread and rice, beans and rice, and almost any stew or pasta sauce served on top of grains accomplishes the same complete amino acid profile.

Protein for Vegetarians

If you're not eating meat or dairy, you will need to work a little harder to eat enough complete protein. There are some vegan protein shakes available with a full spectrum of amino acids.

When you are looking for a high-protein meat substitute, there is nothing that will meet your needs better than tofu. This creamy white product is made from soybeans, nature's *only* complete vegetable protein source. Tofu is extremely bland, causing some people to turn up their noses at it. But the blandness allows tofu to absorb the flavor of other foods, making it easy to cook with.

Not only is tofu an excellent protein source, but it's also low in simple sugars. Always seek out lean proteins and low-fat dairy. In a nutshell (speaking of nuts, they are full of protein), you may eat almost all the lean proteins you like. Protein is a good thing.

As to the Matter of Fat

Protein supplements are also an essential. Lots of varieties exist, so make sure you know what you are looking for! There are formulas with no sugar, no fat or high fat, and with high carbohydrate! This is because many athletes require large amounts of protein to fuel their muscles for sports and find that supplements are a simple, fast source. Some of these athletes require dietary fat, especially if they're trying to gain weight. Others may need the high carbohydrates for endurance. Still others may need a lactose-free product and some contain special nutrient fortifications. If you want to use a protein supplement, choose one with no or low fat, or no sugar.

My nutrition advice in this book focuses on a protein, carbohydrate, and fat balance of 40-40-20. If you want to accelerate weight loss, try to achieve a balance of 50-30-20. Make your portion of lean protein a bit larger than your fist, and your portion of carbohydrates a bit smaller than your fist.

Remember: protein is a good thing. Make it part of every meal.

TAKE THIS THOUGHT TO BED WITH YOU

No, not the book, but this thought for the end of the day!

Everything worthwhile is hardest in the beginning. As your body and mind adapt and you begin to feel better, look better, and enjoy life more, this program gets easier because you're in control. Your body is the most important thing you own—if you don't let it down, it won't let you down!

Have a good night's sleep and feel good. You have accomplished a lot!

Day 1 is finished. Don't forget to pick up with Day 2 first thing in the morning!

Do it! Write it! Be it!

WHAT YOU ATE (If you swallowed it, write it down)

Breakfast: Lunch: Supper:

_____   _____   _____
_____   _____   _____
_____   _____   _____
_____   _____   _____
_____   _____   _____
_____   _____   _____
_____   _____   _____
_____   _____   _____

Snacks:

WHAT YOU DID

Cardiovascular Exercise   Time   Notes

_____   _____   _____
_____   _____   _____

Resistance Exercise   Reps/Sets/Weight   Notes

_____   _____   _____
_____   _____   _____
_____   _____   _____
_____   _____   _____
_____   _____   _____
_____   _____   _____
_____   _____   _____

SUCCESS LOG

DAY 1↑

WHAT YOU THOUGHT

ONLY 27 DAYS TO GO!

DAY 2

BRAIN POWER

Good morning! Start the day with a purpose—and your purpose today is to learn more about how easy it is to make the healthy choices that will improve the way you look, feel, and act! Concentrate on making good choices today. It will pay off!

There are no excuses. We are focused on these 28 days, and getting the maximum results. If you come to a roadblock, just take another road!

EATING RIGHT

Go shopping today and head down the health food aisle of your grocery store or head to the nearest health food store. Stock up on some high-protein, low-carbohydrate prepared meal replacement drinks and/or bars. It can be confusing with so many choices so review the section on page 4 on protein bars and shakes before you go. Pick up a can of protein mix; it will become an essential part of this nutrition plan.

Read the labels and look for protein content per serving of about 19 to 23 grams and carbohydrates of six to ten grams.

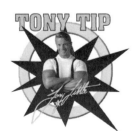

You don't have to weigh or measure your meals or portions. Just keep portion size the same as your closed hand (fist-sized).

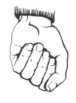

BREAKFAST

Breakfast on the go: Grab a high-protein, low-carbohydrate bar or shake and a low-fat yogurt, preferably plain. Don't forget a vitamin/mineral supplement and water.

Sit-down breakfast: Mix a scoop of protein powder with low-fat, low-sugar yogurt, preferably plain. Also have half a cantaloupe and a slice of whole-grain bread with butter or a trans-fat-free spread. Drink a cup of coffee or tea, black or with a low-fat cream substitute and sugar substitute, if necessary. Or, if you liked it, try the same breakfast as yesterday.

Now head out the door, full steam ahead!

LUNCH

Lunch on the go: Grab a high-protein, low-carbohydrate meal replacement bar, shake, or smoothie. Gobble up a handful of nuts and dried fruit trail mix; stay away from trail mix filled with carob and yogurt chips. Grab one of today's vitamin-enriched water drinks.

Sit-down lunch: Prepare one fist-sized lean hamburger patty, turkey patty, or low-fat veggie burger on a George Foreman grill or fried with Pam. (May be dipped in A-1 sauce or ketchup.) Enjoy with a third of an avocado and half a cup of cottage cheese.

Have an apple or orange for dessert. Drink at least eight ounces of water.

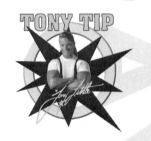

This nutrition plan is not about denial; it's about healthy choices, and there are many. As we progress and you learn more, you can be more creative.

This plan is not designed to starve you! Absolutely not! Starvation is bad, bad, bad, and leads to the rebound effect (yo-yo syndrome) in which you lose muscle, then gain more body fat than before!

This plan is designed to increase your metabolism, promote lean muscle growth, and decrease low-energy body fat. If you're not finding enough carbohydrates you like to eat, go to the list of low-glycemic carbohydrates for alternatives. Life is about choices—good ones and bad ones.

SUPPER

Supper on the go: Hey, you can't have every meal on the go! But if you insist on gulping down a dinner, be smart. A meal replacement shake or smoothie, with a bar, two pieces of fresh fruit, a low-fat, low-sugar yogurt, preferably plain, and plenty of water should tide you over.

Sit-down supper: Grill or bake your choice of flank steak, sole, or tofu scramble or patties. Add a fist-sized portion of green beans, lima beans, spinach, broccoli, bok choy, squash, peas, or salad with oil and vinegar, fat-free Italian dressing, or balsamic vinegar. For your high-energy carbohydrate, try macaroni, risotto, or wild rice.

Again, drink plenty of water. Water helps you lose body fat and it's great for your skin.

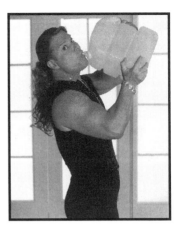

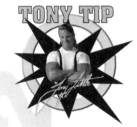

Curb between-meal hunger attacks with a snack of two celery sticks filled with peanut butter. And, if you don't like celery, a teaspoon of peanut butter is awesome!

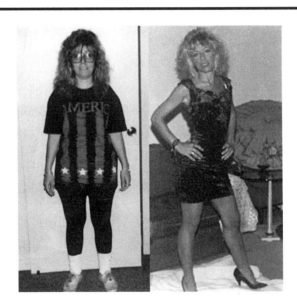

Anna Nicosia from New York lost 27 pounds using Tony's tried-and-true techniques. You can do it too!

WORKOUT

As on every day of this program, we're going to work on our cardio endurance.

Move It or Lose It!
That's a Fact of Life.

We're going to skip resistance exercise today. I know, I know, you're biting at the bit to get into this program 200%, but we're starting out slow and easy, then building up the momentum like that great Tina Turner song "Proud Mary." Now Tina's one chick who knows that keeping it moving keeps you young and rockin'! Just look at her legs and energy levels!

Keep it movin'! Whether it's taking the stairs at a faster pace, jumping up from the couch, or just sprinting to your car, you can find places and times to increase your energy output. Your body was designed to produce energy; work it and it will reward you!

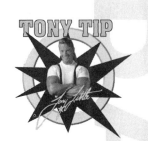

CARDIOVASCULAR EXERCISE

Today we're going to put in 15 minutes of continuous lower body movement—once in the day, once in the evening. Set your watch—and no cheating. It must be continuous!

Pick a different activity than yesterday. Your choices include marching around your living room, stationary cycling, walking outside, walking on a treadmill, gliding on the Gazelle Glider, or using an elliptical machine.

Music is the ultimate motivator—that's why we all tap our feet and move with music. Use it during your cardio sessions and you'll move with more energy. It will also be more fun!

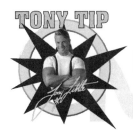

RESISTANCE EXERCISE

Take a break today. We'll get back to our core exercises tomorrow. Instead, do some stretches (see page 301). When was the last time you touched your toes?

Reaching up toward the ceiling, standing on your toes, bending side to side, and performing hip circles are all great ways to awaken your body and keep you limber and flexible. Breathe deeply!

Breathing is important! If you don't do it, you die! But seriously, when you exercise, breathing technique is important. There are two parts to all stretching and resistance exercises: the hard part, and the easy part. For example, in the stretching exercise above, you want to inhale deeply as you reach for the ceiling and stretch, and exhale when you release. In resistance exercise, you want to inhale on the easy part, and exhale on the hard part. So, during an ab crunch, you would exhale on the way up, and inhale on the way down. Breathe deeply. Get that oxygen flowing!

HEALTH SMARTS

METABOLISM: THE KEY TO WEIGHT LOSS AND WHAT DRIVES IT

To effectively lose weight, you must burn off more calories than you consume. A proper diet will reduce your calorie consumption. Exercise will increase the number of calories burned. In order to burn more calories, many people wonder if their time is best spent on cardiovascular exercise or on weight training. To come up with an answer, we've rated the two forms of exercise on the merits of their various benefits.

For fat burning, weights win: Aerobics have long been known as the Queen of Lean. Yes, cardio does indeed burn fat and can definitely contribute to a loss of weight and body fat. But when you stop exercising, you stop burning those calories.

While lifting weights doesn't burn as many calories per minute as cardio, the effort boosts the metabolism, causing you to burn more calories for up to 24 hours after a workout. If you get in a good workout, the total calories burned will be equal to or higher than in cardio. Further, the lean muscle developed burns more calories in maintenance so it's easier to keep the weight off.

For the enjoyment factor, cardio wins: Aerobic dance, kickboxing, or spinning classes provide an excellent support group to get you motivated. Good instructors, of whom there are many, provide the inspiration and incentive to put some real effort into your movements. If you choose individual cardio exercise in a gym, most areas where the treadmills, elliptical trainers, and bicycles are located have TVs, and the time does pass quickly.

Weight training, on the other hand, is an individual sport. It is you against the weight, and some individuals have trouble maintaining the commitment to their workouts and energy needed on their own. It's great for the personal training business, but not so great for the somewhat reluctant exerciser.

For ease of learning, cardio wins: In cardio, you just push a button and go or follow the class instructor. Anyone can learn, in no time.

Weight training is quite a bit more complicated. Routines need to be constantly adjusted for the right benefits, and unless you have excellent guidance to follow, it's very difficult to learn on your own. Weight training also requires learning proper technique to get the maximum benefit: 20 ab crunches properly done go a whole lot further than 50 sloppy ones.

For health benefits, both win: Cardio will increase your lung capacity and aerobic stamina.

Weight training will improve your body composition with more calorie-burning lean muscle. It will improve muscular strength to protect your back and joints. It replaces the natural loss of lean muscle tissue, which begins in the twenties. It helps prevent and repair bone loss from osteoporosis.

An increase in muscle means an increase in metabolism.

For psychological factors, there are benefits to both: Because cardio is usually performed in a separate room from weights, and classes are composed mostly of women, many women find cardio less intimidating than other forms of exercise.

Sometimes a male-dominated weight room can be intimidating. But today many women-only clubs are opening and expanding. Also, not all women are intimidated by men's weight rooms; some love weight training for that very reason! Of course, as with cardio, you can always train at home.

The answer: As you can see, both forms of exercise are equally crucial to your health. You can be lean, mean, and strong as an ox, but if you don't have any lung capacity, you still won't be able to swim a lap or make it to the top of a long flight of stairs without panting. The bottom line: you need them both.

If you're exercising to combat the effects of aging, it's more important than ever to hit the weight room. Lean muscle and growth hormones decline with age, causing energy and strength to diminish and fat stores to increase. Weight training is a veritable fountain of youth. A healthy weight-trained physique will also do much to improve posture, balance, and mobility. Use your cardio as a warm-up for the weight routine, just as it is used in this program.

What you eat also affects your metabolism. Follow the healthy eating plan in this book along with the exercise program and you'll be increasing your metabolism while burning calories to the max. The combo can't be beat.

TAKE THIS THOUGHT TO BED WITH YOU

Life is full of choices. Today you've made some healthy ones. Congratulations! I'm sure you've made some bad choices in the past that have adversely affected your energy level and well-being (haven't we all?), but for the next few weeks, it's positive, it's good, and you're in control.

Sleep well. This is the time when your body regenerates and replenishes. Let it work its magic.

Day 2, finished!

Do it! Write it! Be it!

WHAT YOU ATE (If you swallowed it, write it down)

Breakfast: Lunch: Supper:

_____   _____   _____
_____   _____   _____
_____   _____   _____
_____   _____   _____
_____   _____   _____
_____   _____   _____
_____   _____   _____

Snacks:

WHAT YOU DID

Cardiovascular Exercise   Time   Notes

_____   _____   _____
_____   _____   _____

Resistance Exercise   Reps/Sets/Weight   Notes

_____   _____   _____
_____   _____   _____
_____   _____   _____
_____   _____   _____
_____   _____   _____
_____   _____   _____
_____   _____   _____

WHAT YOU THOUGHT

_____
_____
_____
_____
_____
_____
_____
_____
_____
_____
_____
_____
_____
_____
_____
_____
_____
_____
_____
_____
_____
_____
_____
_____
_____
_____

DAY 2

ONLY 26 DAYS TO GO!

DAY 3

BRAIN POWER

Time counts.

Imagine if every day you were given $1,440 that you could spend any way you wanted. The only downside is that if you didn't spend it all, the balance would be gone when you woke up. But, you would get another $1,440 to start all over again.

What would you do? Most people would try to squeeze every last red cent out of their daily allotment. Right?

There are 1,440 minutes in each day, and what you don't use, you lose. Make certain you get the most out of every single second of those minutes. Time counts; use it or lose it!

EATING RIGHT

Consider a cup of apple chunks or slices for a between-meal snack. It satisfies, without the fat or calories, and offers high energy.

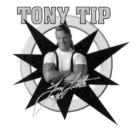

Search for a balance in your food choices. This keeps your energy up and your insulin on an even keel. Aim to get 40% of your calories from protein, 40% from carbohydrates, and 20% from fat. For enhanced weight loss benefits, try a plan of 50% protein, 30% carbohydrates, and 20% fat.

BREAKFAST

Breakfast on the go: Grab a fruit cup and a low-fat, low-sugar yogurt, preferably plain, or a high-protein, low-carbohydrate smoothie or bar.

Sit-down breakfast: Have one toasted whole-wheat bagel with a little reduced-fat cream cheese. Top with lox, sardines, smoked salmon, or a slice of deli meat with a slice of tomato. Or, have eggs or egg substitute on the bagel. You can have one cup of coffee or tea, black or with a low-fat cream substitute and sugar substitute, if necessary.

LUNCH

Lunch on the go: Have a high-protein, low-carbohydrate shake, smoothie, or bar. Add a piece of fresh fruit or raw celery, broccoli or carrots. If that's too little too soon for you, reach for a tuna or peanut butter and jam (all fruit, no sugar added) sandwich on whole-grain bread. Drink plenty of water.

Sit-down lunch: Turn to the back of the book for some quick recipes, like our quick chili with a fist-sized portion of diced veal, chicken, or lean beef; celery; green pepper; mushrooms; and kidney beans. Add a spoonful of salsa and some canned tomatoes. Have an apple or orange for dessert and drink plenty of water.

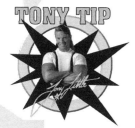

Always keep a good stock of fresh fruit and prepared drinks and meal replacement bars. Keep the drinks cold in your refrigerator, ready to grab as you head out the door.

SUPPER

Supper on the go: Go for that meal replacement bar or shake. Have fresh fruit and a hard-boiled egg (available at most deli counters) on the side. Drink plenty of water, water, water.

Sit-down supper: Simple. Choose a fist-sized piece of lean meat, and from the list of low-glycemic carbohydrates, select a fist-sized portion of vegetables (yellow, green, or red) and a fist-size portiond of carbohydrates, plus one piece of fruit.

Always drink plenty of water with your meals.

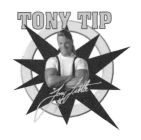

Take small bites and eat slowly. Keep portions the size of your fist. Don't aim for full, aim for satisfied! Do not eat for two to three hours before you go to sleep. Remember, four or five small meals daily will help you lose weight fast while maintaining the muscle for shape and calorie burning.

WORKOUT

Yep, you're catching on! Cardio rules! You should include it as a regular part of your fitness routine forever! If possible, mornings are best. We will also go back to conditioning our core body strength area: abs, back, and legs.

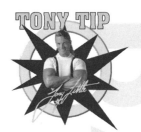

Cardio five days a week! Remember cardio can come in many forms: a walk through the shopping mall on Saturday, a bicycle ride, hiking with the kids or dog, or an evening dancing. Get your cardio when you can—just keep it continuous and low impact!

CARDIOVASCULAR EXERCISE

We're looking for just 20 minutes of continuous cardio today!

Choices of exercises include marching around your living room, stationary cycling, walking or jogging, walking on a treadmill, gliding on the Gazelle Glider, or using the elliptical machine. No need to check heart rate yet. Brisk movement is the key.

> ## Be sure to write down your exercise and meals!

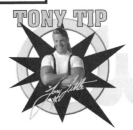

The more body parts you move, the better the workout and the more calories burned.

RESISTANCE EXERCISE

Progressive resistance exercise, as the story goes, began in Greece when a farm boy named Milo began to lift his baby cow into the back of a wagon. Over time as the calf grew, the boy's strength also grew, until he was able to lift the small cow into the wagon. Of course, you don't have to lift a cow, just some weights, which will get progressively heavier.

That's how we're going to do it, adding just a little more work to each workout, while giving you time to recuperate from the one before.

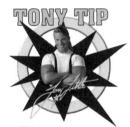

Cardio exercise works the fastest to help you burn calories and lose weight. Resistance training takes longer, but its effect is greater because it builds lean muscle mass, which in turn increases your metabolism to burn more calories throughout the day—even while at rest!

Tony's Squeeze and Stretch Technique Spells Success!

Always, when performing any resistance exercise, employ Tony's Squeeze and Stretch Technique. Put your mental muscle to work and *squeeze* the muscle you're working (plus all the other muscles that assist) while you perform the weighted portion of any exercise. This is like an isometric movement, which employs both the muscle being worked and its opposing muscle group. Thus, in performing a biceps curl, you squeeze the biceps and also receive benefit to the triceps.

---

1. Ab crunch (midsection):

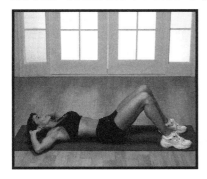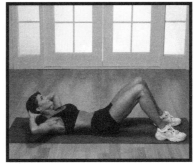

When you crunch, think *squeeze!* Lie on your back with your knees bent as shown. Place your whole back to the floor, leaving no space between you and the floor. Keep your chin up. Keep your eyes to the ceiling. Place your hands lightly against your head. Roll your shoulders forward, bringing your head toward your knees. Keep your lower back on the floor, feet planted solidly.

Throughout this exercise, keep the muscles of your abs and buttocks tense. At the peak of the crunch, exhale and *squeeze* even harder, slowly and precisely.

SET ONE: 10–15 repetitions
SET TWO: 10–15 repetitions

2. Reverse crunch (midsection):

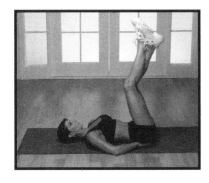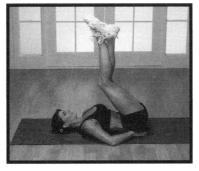

This exercise works the lower portion of the abs. Lie with your hands under your lower back (as shown). Think *squeeze* and send a mental message to make all the muscles of your torso tense. With your legs together, knees slightly bent, slowly rock your knees up toward your shoulders, being careful not to allow your lower back to leave the mat. Think technique!

SET ONE: 10–15 repetitions
SET TWO: 10–15 repetitions

3. Lying back extension (lower back):

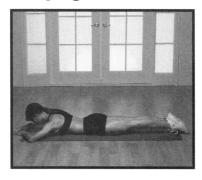 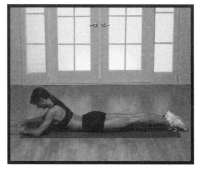

Always work your lower back when you work your abs. Lie face down on a mat or towel on the floor. Place your arms in front of you (as shown). Keeping your legs straight, push your upper torso off the floor. This is similar to the Cobra move in Tai Chi. Really *squeeze* at this point and hold for one second before repeating.

SET ONE: 10–15 repetitions
SET TWO: 10–15 repetitions

4. One-half squats (front and back of upper legs):

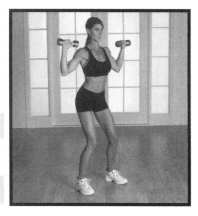 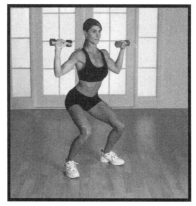

Strong legs support core strength, and the squat is the king of the leg exercises. We'll begin with a one-half squat. Use your own bodyweight or light, 5- to 15-pound dumbbells. With feet shoulder-width apart, stand as shown. Hold dumbbells as shown or resting lightly on shoulders. Slowly squat down as though you were about to sit in a chair. Go only halfway down, and push with your legs back up to a standing position.

SET ONE: 10–15 repetitions
SET TWO: 10–15 repetitions

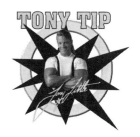

When you're just beginning an exercise program after a long time off, it's important that you rest for at least one full minute between sets. Stop exercising immediately if you feel faint or lightheaded. Always stretch before and after a workout.

That's the way to do it! You've now accomplished twice the work from Day 1. We've already doubled the workload. Just think what your conditioning level is going to be at the end of the program!

Want More?

It's okay to add some daily stretches, perform extra reps, or sneak in an extra cardio session. But don't push yourself too hard—it's only Day 3! As with the tortoise and the hare, slow and easy wins this race.

HEALTH SMARTS

THE TEN MOST IMPORTANT STEPS TO LOSING WEIGHT AND KEEPING IT OFF

1. Choose lean protein such as eggs, egg substitutes, lean beef, turkey, chicken, fish, or tofu for vegetarians. Only broil, bake, boil, or poach. Use only olive oil or Pam spray.
2. Minimize consumption of high-glycemic carbohydrates (carbohydrates that make your blood sugar level spike) such as white rice, sugar, certain pastas, and potatoes. Seek out cereals that are low glycemic for good-body choices. (See chart on page 5.)
3. When eating carbohydrates, eat them with proteins and keep the portion size small.
4. Eat high-fiber foods or add fiber to your diet.
5. Water, water, water. Drink lots of water daily. Drink it before a meal to help get you more full quickly.
6. Try and stay with 40% protein, 40% carbohydrate, 20% fat within your food sources. (Change this to 50% protein, 30% carbohydrate, and 20% fat when

you are trying to lose weight)

7. Eat four to six small meals a day, or a meal replacement bar for one of the meals.

8. Portion sizes of everything should be the size of your fist. The amount of protein can be increased if you are exercising intensely.

9. When eating out, remember to have your food cooked the right way. After all, you are the one paying. Limit condiments on your food and you will actually begin to notice the quality of the meal.

10. Do cardio exercise at least 30 to 45 minutes three to five times a week. Do resistance exercise with weights or machines for 20 to 30 minutes two or three times a week, using mostly large muscle groups to speed your metabolism.

TAKE THIS THOUGHT TO BED WITH YOU

Of your 1,440 minutes today, how many did you put to a good, productive, and positive use? All that you had available? That's great. Use the rest wisely to have a pleasant night's sleep. Rest is as important as work in a healthy lifestyle.

Dream big; there's no use wasting minutes on little dreams. And remember, whatever you conceive, and believe, you can achieve.

Pleasant dreams!

Day 3 finished. See you in the morning.

Do it! Write it! Be it!

WHAT YOU ATE (If you swallowed it, write it down)

Breakfast: Lunch: Supper:

_____   _____   _____
_____   _____   _____
_____   _____   _____
_____   _____   _____
_____   _____   _____
_____   _____   _____
_____   _____   _____
_____   _____   _____

Snacks:

WHAT YOU DID

Cardiovascular Exercise   Time   Notes

_____   _____   _____
_____   _____   _____

Resistance Exercise   Reps/Sets/Weight   Notes

_____   _____   _____
_____   _____   _____
_____   _____   _____
_____   _____   _____
_____   _____   _____
_____   _____   _____
_____   _____   _____

WHAT YOU THOUGHT

_____
_____
_____
_____
_____
_____
_____
_____
_____
_____
_____
_____
_____
_____
_____
_____
_____
_____
_____
_____
_____
_____
_____
_____
_____
_____
_____
_____

ONLY 25 DAYS TO GO!

DAY 31

DAY 4

BRAIN POWER

It's our hump day! You're halfway through your first week. You've done well, but the best is yet to come.

Take a quick assessment of the many healthy food choices you've made this week and of your start of a great exercise program. I knew you could do it, and now it's time to give yourself a pat on the back.

Why not treat yourself to something special today like a long bath, a pedicure, a soothing massage, or a romantic, candlelit evening with your favorite person?

My one-on-one program involves some work, but it also involves rewards. Reward yourself often and generously. (This doesn't mean a huge piece of chocolate cake!)

EATING RIGHT

Eating well is about making healthy choices. The adjustments you've made in your meals thus far are beginning to have an effect on your body.

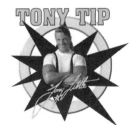

Should you get on the scale? Sure, you may take a base weight, but don't get fixated on the numbers. There are so many other things happening in your body that weight loss on the scale may not show up for weeks.

Instead, use that article of clothing you picked out earlier that did not fit, and try that on when you want to see if there is a change. You'll notice this program works first on your body proportions, and second on your overall weight.

Record workouts and meals!
This is very important!

BREAKFAST

Breakfast on the go: Mix canned fruit with low-fat cottage cheese and have a vitamin/mineral supplement.

Sit-down breakfast: Pam-fry some egg whites, egg substitute, or tofu with diced vegetables. Have this with rye or pumpernickel bread with a healthy spread, one piece of fruit, and plenty of water.

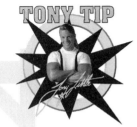

Curb the cravings with a choice from the following high-energy snacks: an ounce of lean deli meat, ten almonds and one medium apple, or one hard-boiled egg.

LUNCH

Lunch on the go: Order a fist-sized portion of lean deli meat on rye or pumpernickel bread with mustard, no mayonnaise, and all the vegetables you like. Drink as much water as you can drink.

Sit-down lunch: Brown a fist-sized portion of lean ground turkey, drain the fat, and mix with some premade pasta sauce. Spoon over cooked whole-wheat pasta noodles and enjoy with steamed vegetables with reduced-fat butter and lemon.

Have fruit for dessert. Drink at least eight ounces of water.

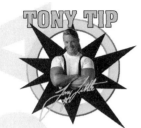

This lunch recipe is a perfect example of something you can prepare the night before and have a sit-down meal reheated in on-the-go time!

SUPPER

Supper on the go: Have a meal replacement shake or bar or head down to Subway for one of their six-inch, under-six-grams-of-fat sandwiches. Drink plenty of water.

Sit-down supper: Choose a fist-sized portion of lean meat, a fist-sized portion of fresh or frozen vegetables, a fist-sized portion of low-glycemic carbohydrates from our list, plus one piece of fruit. Or check the recipes in the back of the book. Always drink plenty of water with your meals.

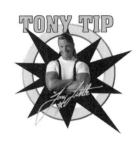

Obey your hunger. Eat when you're hungry. Stop eating when you're satisfied. There is no such thing as the Clean Plate Club and there is no way to send the food you don't eat off to a third-world country to feed starving children. Don't overeat, no matter what!

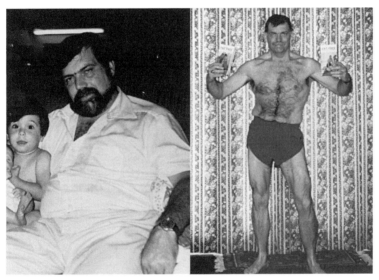

*Weight loss isn't just a woman's problem.
Chuck Toles from New York lost a whopping 97 pounds!
He did it! You can do it!*

EXERCISE

It's another 15 minutes of cardio—and that's four days in a row! If you've found a favorite activity, repeat it. Check the time and keep it moving for a full 15 minutes. If you feel you're ready, put a little more energy into today's workouts than you did yesterday.

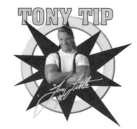

You don't need to take your heart rate. Right now using the Perceived Rate of Exertion (PRE) scale will work fine. Imagine yourself chased by a pack of slobbering, growling, fang-snapping wolves and running as fast as your legs will carry you. That's an 11 on the scale—and we don't want to go there! Not yet!

On the other side of the scale is walking, which is a 3. Watching TV is a 0. Walking upstairs is about a 4.5.

Depending on your current level of conditioning, you should be performing your cardio at a PRE of between 4 and 6.

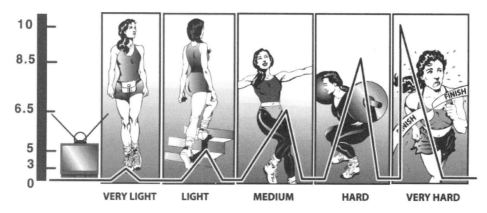

Perceived Exertion Chart
Illustration by Matt Gouig

CARDIOVASCULAR EXERCISE

Do you have a favorite exercise video, maybe one of mine? You might try finding a 15-minute segment performed at the proper tempo and use that today for a change of pace. Perform two 15-minute sessions today—one in the day, one in the evening. You can mix them up: you don't have to perform the same routine twice. Choose from the bike, treadmill, elliptical trainer, or Gazelle Glider.

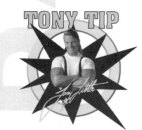

If you feel you're getting too tired, take the Talk Test. Try to carry on a normal conversation for 30 seconds. If you have to gasp, you're working too hard. Cut back immediately!

RESISTANCE EXERCISE

You get a break from your resistance exercise again today. Take some time for a couple of basic stretches (see page 301), and seek out a way to burn some extra calories, like skipping around the house, doing a quick set of jumping jacks, or lying on your back and air cycling!

Those activities are what athletes call "active rest."

Make a habit of inserting active rests into your spare time. It will put a lift in your step and a song in your heart. Plus, your body will look better!

HEALTH SMARTS

NEED SOME MOTIVATION? LOOK IN THE MIRROR!

What stands between you and your good health is not the lack of a program or advice on proper nutrition. There are hundreds of great programs and thousands of supplements, bars, shakes, snacks, and drinks to ensure you receive optimum nutrition.

What's stopping you?

It may be motivation. Tomorrow is always a better time to start a new diet. Next week you'll start that Tae Boxing class you've heard so much about. And you know that you shouldn't have seconds of that creamy, rich, fresh-from-the-oven chocolate fudge brownie, but what the heck? One more won't do that much harm, and besides, you're going to start that diet and exercise program any day now, right?

So it goes until your weight balloons, your cholesterol and blood pressure rise and your blood sugar begins alternately to spike and plummet. You are now officially overweight and out of shape.

Good Intentions . . . But

Some people manage to maintain a healthy weight and nutritious diet without any problem. Most of us do not. When the years begin to steal our youthful vitality, many of us sit back and let nature take its worst course.

Most all of us resolve at many times to make our lifestyles healthier. New Year's is the perfect example: 80% of us resolve each year to begin a healthier diet and lifestyle. The health club industry does more than 50% of its entire year's business in the first three months of the year. It is also estimated that the dropout rate is higher than 50% in the first six months.

A Bad Pattern

Other than padding the pockets of health club owners, our yearly cycle of promising to live healthier then discontinuing because of frustration over our own inconsistency just breeds more of the same! When people do not succeed, they view themselves as failures or resort to rationalizations like "I don't have the time" or "I have more important things to do" or "I'll do it tomorrow." So it goes in a circle of resolution and disillusion.

Breaking the Cycle

I believe that this is the perfect program to finally meet those goals that have only been wishes until now. The program is new to you, but its methods have already worked for tens of thousands of people. And everything is spelled out, day by day. But you need the proper mind-set or philosophical approach in order to accomplish your goals. Also, after this program, if you ever hit a sticking point, remember *variety is key!* Change exercises around, switch days, and so on.

Always believe it's now or never in your mind.

No matter what kind of shape you're in, success is first achieved in your mind! Start there; the rest will follow.

Small Steps

Achievements are a process. You don't luck out on them; you work systematically toward them. Your good health should be seen as an achievement you will consciously make.

Begin by setting small, realistic, and clearly defined goals. Good health is a byproduct of healthy lifestyle habits. Illness and a life cut unnecessarily short are often the result of unhealthy lifestyle habits. To change a habit, you need to mentally commit to the process, then incrementally take the small steps to instill new, healthy habits.

What Goes Wrong

People fail at their goals because they do not have a clear plan. A wish is just a wish; a goal is something that can be achieved and that has attached to it a clear methodology to achieve the goal.

As I've said before, a wish means nothing. A decision means everything. Your decision to do this program will change your life. I promise.

Another reason people fail is that they set their expectations too high. Be reasonable. Make a plan of incremental steps. Then take it one day at a time, but always with your goal and those steps clearly in mind at the start of each day.

The biggest reason people fail is that they fear the unknown. Unless you are armed with information about optimal nutrition and exercise, you will never have enough faith in your plan to carry it out. Action is key to achievement. Education is key to finding the winning course of action. So, to sum it up, set a goal; make a clear, realistic plan; and make a decision to accomplish the goal in a realistic time period. Chart your progress and have regular goal assessment and progress meetings with yourself!

Day 4, done. Rest up for the morning. And by the way, great job. You're no slob!

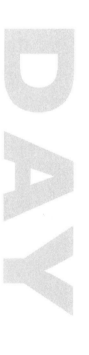

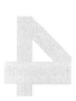

Do it! Write it! Be it!

WHAT YOU ATE (If you swallowed it, write it down)

Breakfast: Lunch: Supper:

_____   _____   _____
_____   _____   _____
_____   _____   _____
_____   _____   _____
_____   _____   _____
_____   _____   _____
_____   _____   _____
_____   _____   _____

Snacks:

WHAT YOU DID

Cardiovascular Exercise   Time   Notes

_____   _____   _____
_____   _____   _____

Resistance Exercise   Reps/Sets/Weight   Notes

_____   _____   _____
_____   _____   _____
_____   _____   _____
_____   _____   _____
_____   _____   _____
_____   _____   _____
_____   _____   _____

WHAT YOU THOUGHT

ONLY 24 DAYS TO GO!

DAY 5

Balance in your life is important—for the inside and outside.

Think of your inner balance as if you were riding a bicycle. On a bicycle, you must maintain balance and keep moving to stay upright. In life, you must stay even-tempered to avoid stress and stay healthy.

Look today for five disappointments, losses, or missed opportunities. When you encounter each of them, just keep on pedaling at your own comfortable pace. Don't let those inevitable things get you down. You are on the fast track to success, and keep that at the forefront of your mind. You'll smile at the end of the day.

EATING RIGHT

Be honest. Did you think you'd make it to Day 5 this easily? Try to follow day by day, but if you need to be more creative, check out the list for more low-glycemic food choices and the back of the book for more one-on-one recipes.

BREAKFAST

Breakfast on the go: Nothing beats a high-protein, low-carbohydrate shake in the morning with a piece of fruit, a vitamin/mineral supplement, and water.

Sit-down breakfast: Prepare three eggs (or egg substitute or egg whites), poached, fried with Pam spray, or scrambled. On the side, have two slices of whole-grain bread with an all-fruit, no-sugar spread. One cup of coffee or tea, no sugar, black or with a low-fat cream substitute. You may also have a six-ounce glass of orange juice. Try to eat the fruit and bread before the eggs, if possible.

LUNCH

Lunch on the go: Grab that high-protein, low-carbohydrate smoothie or bar. Be sure to drink plenty of water with lunch and throughout the day!

Keep your on-the-go meal replacement bars to no more than two a day. You may choose ready-to-drink smoothies and shakes and keep a stockpile in your fridge. Or you may mix your own with ice, water, or nonfat milk and a high-protein, low-carbohydrate powder.

Sit-down lunch: Salad always works. Add a small amount of reduced-fat mayonnaise or salad dressing to a six- or eight-ounce can of water-packed tuna. Mix with peas and/or chopped celery and spread onto two slices of whole-wheat or whole-grain bread for a high-protein, low-carbohydrate lunch. Hint: add a little mustard or pickle relish to moisten your tuna salad.

If you don't like tuna, try a chicken breast—grilled, baked, or broiled without the skin—on two slices of bread with lettuce, tomato, and mayonnaise. Turkey is also okay as long as it's breast meat.

Have an apple or orange for dessert. Drink at least eight ounces of water.

SUPPER

Supper on the go: Drink a high-protein, low-carbohydrate smoothie or shake, or eat one high-protein, low-carbohydrate bar. Add a hard-boiled egg and a piece of fruit, and be sure to drink eight ounces or more of water!

Sit-down supper: Friday is grill time! Grill or broil a fist-sized cube steak patty (you may substitute tuna steak, salmon, chicken breast, or turkey), and add a fist-sized portion of green beans, lima beans, spinach, or salad with oil and vinegar, fat-free Italian dressing, or balsamic vinegar. Have one sweet or baked potato with light butter or trans-fat-free spread (read the label). Try a bit of A-1 sauce on your potato!

Again, drink plenty of water. Water helps you lose body fat and it is great for your skin, as well as for bad backs. Staying hydrated is good for all the joints of the body. Remember, a hydrated body is a happier body!

WORKOUT

Today we do cardio and core exercises—both with more power, enthusiasm, and results!

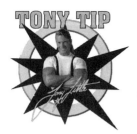

CARDIOVASCULAR EXERCISE

You've built up a little arsenal of cardio routines. Pick one and invest 25 minutes of your time. Remember to work at a PRE of 4 to 7. Remember, a PRE (Perceived Rate of Exertion) of 0 is the effort you put out to watch TV. A PRE of 3 is like vacuuming the carpet. A PRE of 10 is like running to save not only your life, but also the lives of your child, parents, and partner. Today's PRE of 4 to 7 means some effort!

Music will help the time go faster. Plus, regular cardio exercise reduces day-to-day stress that can sabotage your efforts!

Be sure to keep track of everything!

RESISTANCE EXERCISE

We're adding a third set to our core routine. Strive to do the recommended reps and sets. But if you fall a little short, don't sweat it.

Resistance exercise takes work. It's the effort that separates resistance exercise from cardio. On your PRE scale, you want to be working between a 4 and a 7. That means you might let a little grunt or groan escape you. That's good!

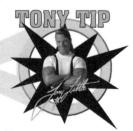

On a three-set program, a challenging routine can be described as one that allows you to complete the prescribed reps in the first set, barely complete them in the second set, and fall a little short on the third set, if you have to. If it gets easier than this, increase your weights, or your repetitions.

The number of sets and reps are only recommendations. If you ever feel faint or lightheaded, stop immediately. At this point, allow a one-minute rest between your sets.

1. Ab crunch (midsection):

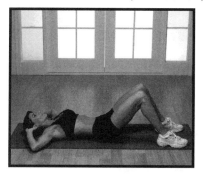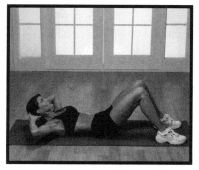

When you crunch, think *squeeze!* Lie on your back with your knees bent as shown. Keep your chin up. Keep your eyes to the ceiling. Place your hands lightly against the sides of your head. Roll your shoulders forward, bringing your head toward your knees. Keep your lower back on the floor, feet planted solidly.

Throughout this exercise, keep the muscles of your abs and buttocks tense. At the peak of the crunch, exhale and *squeeze* even harder, slowly and precisely.

SET ONE: 10–15 repetitions
SET TWO: 10–15 repetitions
SET THREE: 10–15 repetitions

2. Reverse crunch (midsection):

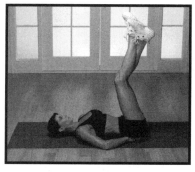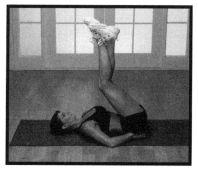

This exercise works the lower portion of the abs. Lie with your hands under your lower back (as shown). Think *squeeze* and send a mental message to make all the muscles of your torso tense. With your legs together, knees slightly bent, slowly rock your knees up toward your shoulders, being careful not to allow your lower back to leave the mat. Think technique!

SET ONE: 10–15 repetitions
SET TWO: 10–15 repetitions
SET THREE: 10–15 repetitions

DAY 5

3. Lying back extension (lower back):

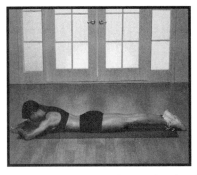 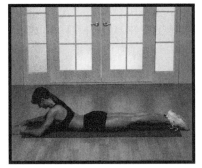

Always work your lower back when you work your abs. Lie face down on a mat or towel on the floor. Place your arms in front of you (as shown). Keeping your legs straight, push your upper torso off the floor. Really *squeeze* your glutes and hamstrings at this point and hold for one second before repeating.

SET ONE: 10–15 repetitions
SET TWO: 10–15 repetitions
SET THREE: 10–15 repetitions

4. One-half squat (front and back of upper legs):

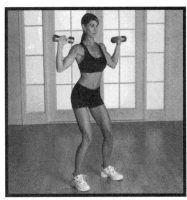 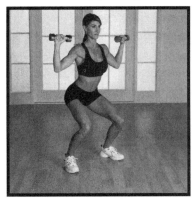

Strong legs support core strength, and the squat is the king of the leg exercises. We'll begin with a one-half squat. Use your bodyweight or light, 5- to 15-pound dumbbells. With feet shoulder-width apart, stand as shown. *Squeeze.* Hold dumbbells as shown or resting lightly on shoulders. Slowly squat down as though you were about to sit in a chair. Go only halfway down, and push with your legs back up to a standing position.

SET ONE: 10–15 repetitions
SET TWO: 10–15 repetitions
SET THREE: 8–12 repetitions

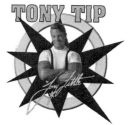

If you've got the energy to complete more reps, go for it! Those extra reps are always the ones that count the most!

You have now completed your circuit of core strength exercises. Spend the rest of the day walking just a little taller, proud of your accomplishment. And take a moment to listen to your body . . . it likes what you're doing, doesn't it?

Now while you're at it, think about posture. Sit tall. Walk tall. Eventually it will become a habit and it will add to your fitness.

HEALTH SMARTS

THE SCALE IS PUBLIC ENEMY NO. 1

If I could, I'd take all the personal body weight scales and toss them out! Scales are not effective at measuring healthy weight loss.

I can't tell you how many times I've heard people lament that the four pounds they lost at home all came back at the doctor's office. Come on, the weight didn't come back; it's just that most scales are not accurate, and your weight fluctuates throughout the day. You can actually lose significant body fat, and it won't necessarily show on the scale if you've gained some lean muscle at the same time!

The opposite holds true as well. You can lose weight in an unhealthy fashion, and it will show on the scale, but your body starts to look like a skeleton with loose skin draped upon it!

It's In Your Head

Many people get so obsessed with their morning weigh-in that it sets the theme for the entire day. A few pounds up and they start the day feeling fat, sluggish, and with a what's-the-use attitude toward their workout and diet.

Come on, folks, we don't need that!

There are many factors affecting scale weight. Let's start with the fact that home-use scales are not always calibrated correctly. Many scales will weigh you differently if you stand at the front, or back, or to one side or another. The time of day affects what the scale says.

Now, consider this. Wrestling, bodybuilding, or other weight class events have specific weigh-ins. It is usually in the best interest of the athlete to weigh in at the top of their class. It is not uncommon at these weigh-ins to see athletes standing on their heads. Why? Because a few minutes on your head will cause the scale to read you several pounds lighter!

So if you work your heart out to please the scale, you may be getting false signals—either good or bad.

The best way to assess healthy weight loss is the tape measure. You should have taken your measurements the first day, and written them down. Now, take them again and write them down. Check page 8 for the proper body points to measure. Keep this up throughout the program. That's where you will see in inches how your hard work paid off.

Another easy way to measure the change in your body is to use that pair of pants, shorts, or even shirt that you can barely fit into without busting the seams or buttons. The fit should be such that you can get it on, but can't move or breathe in it. Set that garment aside, and periodically throughout this program try it on again. You might be surprised at how quickly your body reproportions itself!

Body fat testing is not as easy to do, but also a good method to check your results. This one-on-one program is not after a simple loss of pounds as healthy pounds make a body look great. We want to lose the fat. Some health clubs have the test available for a low cost. Your physician can also order a very accurate test. Skin calipers, used by a professional, are also a form of body fat testing. Try to do this very soon, and then again at the end. You'll see the results!

Whatever methods you use, please, please don't use that dang scale!

TAKE THIS THOUGHT TO BED WITH YOU

Before you fall asleep, make a mental checklist of your body, from head to toe. Now, follow your checklist, relaxing each part as you go. Are your toes relaxed, ankles, shins, knees, and quads? Good. Now keep going up your body until every inch of you is relaxed and comfortable.

Remind yourself how good it feels to be in your body. Congratulate yourself on working to make yourself feel even better in the skin you're in.

Pleasant dreams.

Do it! Write it! Be it!

WHAT YOU ATE (If you swallowed it, write it down)

Breakfast: Lunch: Supper:

_____   _____   _____
_____   _____   _____
_____   _____   _____
_____   _____   _____
_____   _____   _____
_____   _____   _____
_____   _____   _____

Snacks:

WHAT YOU DID

Cardiovascular Exercise   Time   Notes

_____   _____   _____
_____   _____   _____

Resistance Exercise   Reps/Sets/Weight   Notes

_____   _____   _____
_____   _____   _____
_____   _____   _____
_____   _____   _____
_____   _____   _____
_____   _____   _____
_____   _____   _____
_____   _____   _____

WHAT YOU THOUGHT

_____
_____
_____
_____
_____
_____
_____
_____
_____
_____
_____
_____
_____
_____
_____
_____
_____
_____
_____
_____
_____
_____
_____
_____
_____
_____
_____
_____

ONLY 23 DAYS TO GO!

DAY 6

BRAIN POWER

Five days out of each week you should treat your body as a temple—with respect and reverence. Two days out of the week you should treat your body as an amusement park—with wonder, excitement, and joy. Welcome to your amusement day. Maybe you should go to an amusement park. Enjoy today to its fullest.

EATING RIGHT

Hey, it's the weekend, so you may find yourself making some modifications. That's okay. Refer to the list of low-glycemic carbohydrates, and be creative!

BREAKFAST

Breakfast on the go: Grab a high-protein, low-carbohydrate meal replacement bar or drink, some fresh fruit, and a bottle of water as you head out the door!

Sit-down breakfast: Try half a cup of slow-cooked oats (or low-fat, low-sodium, high-fiber cereal) with berries, nuts, and fat-free milk. Also have a scoop of protein powder mixed with low-fat yogurt, preferably plain, and a slice of whole-grain bread with butter or a trans-fat-free spread. For a drink, have a cup of coffee or tea, no sugar, black or with a low-fat cream substitute.

You're loaded with high-energy carbohydrates and slow-burning protein, so head out the door, full steam ahead!

LUNCH

Lunch on the go: Try one of Subway's six-inch, under-six-grams-of-fat sandwiches or a healthy meal replacement bar or shake. Or, go to a deli and get a sandwich of turkey or chicken breast on whole wheat or grain bread—no cheese. Ask them to go light on the mayonnaise! As usual, don't forget the water!

Sit-down lunch: Make a couple of bean burritos with extra lettuce or go out for a chunky chicken salad, fajita salad, or Cobb salad without the bacon. Use no more than two tablespoons of dressing.

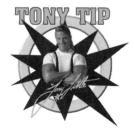

Instead of asking for dressing on the side, then pouring it on your salad, dip your fork in the dressing, and then put some salad on your fork. You will be surprised how little dressing you actually need!

SUPPER

Supper on the go: Have a high-protein, low-carbohydrate meal replacement shake with extra fresh fruit and a handful of unsalted walnuts and almonds, plus lots of water.

Sit-down supper: Check the list of low-glycemic carbohydrates and choose a lean meat or protein source, vegetables, and a carbohydrate, then fix proper proportions for yourself and enjoy. Or, take yourself out to a restaurant and request selections from your list. You'd be surprised to find out how willing most restaurants are to please you.

Always drink plenty of water with your meals. Sorbet or fruit and cheese for dessert are great.

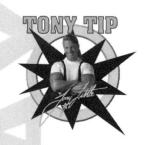

Eating out doesn't mean you eat whatever they serve you. Be bold and request meats broiled or grilled, not fried; vegetables should be steamed, not boiled; and portions can be served plain, without the rich sauces. It's your body; it's your choice.

And if the portions are too large, request the to-go box at the beginning of the meal and spoon what's more than a fistful off your plate before you have a chance to eat it.

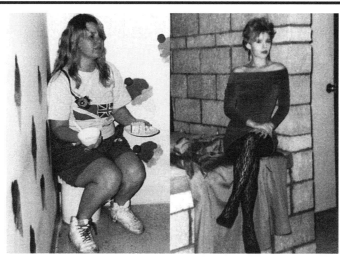

Weight loss comes to those who stick with it,
like Pattie Simon from Florida who lost 60 pounds!
Congratulations, Pattie!

WORKOUT

We're going to make today a day of active rest! There is no formal exercise, but don't forget to keep your body moving! Take some time today to stretch. You can check out page 301 for stretching ideas, but come on, we all know how to do it! Try to stretch for 15 minutes today!

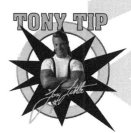

Look for creative ways to get some extra cardio in today. What about a hike or a bike ride with a friend or your pet? Rollerblades, anyone? How about putting on those headphones and heading outside, if you haven't already?

RESISTANCE EXERCISE

No core exercises today, but put my active rest plan to use. Do some chores around the house that have you stretching and lifting (cleaning closets and garages always seem to provide this) or go outside in your garden. Rake some fall leaves, shovel some winter snow, plant some spring flowers, or prune some summer foliage. Remember, when lifting from the floor or ground, use your legs, not your back!

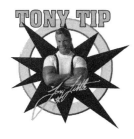

TONY TIP

Do something you haven't done in a long time. When was the last time you skated, cycled, played a game of tennis, played softball, bowled, or went for a swim?

Look back and find some physical activity you used to love, and renew it. Even if you go at it at a slower pace, you'll rediscover the same love that you had for it before.

Think young today, all day long. You can do it!

HEALTH SMARTS

SUPERSIZE IT, AND YOU'LL SUPERSIZE YOURSELF!

Excuse me while I climb on my soapbox. It's great to have food prepared your way, but don't make it the fast-food way! Fast food is largely responsible for the epidemic of obesity in America. Fast food is also largely responsible for the rising rates of heart disease and diabetes we have in this country.

Fast food has literally changed the way people eat. Europeans laugh at us for being a nation on the run, dashing through the drive-thru window and gobbling down a triple-deluxe burger as we careen down the highway. Personally, I prefer to dine at home with mellow music. Eating, for me, is one of life's great pleasures.

Far worse than indigestion from scarfing fast food is the nutritional makeup of these foods. Sure, they contain protein, and protein is good for us. Unfortunately, protein content is the only good thing I can see in fast food.

Fast food is loaded with simple high-glycemic carbohydrates that not only are stored as fat but also contribute to food cravings, bingeing, and diabetes. Fast food is chock-full of fat and sodium, and very low in fiber. Further, consuming fast food crowds out fresh fruits and vegetables, milk, and other nutrient-packed foods from our diets.

Fast food is a huge, rich, and powerful industry. Although the industry has been pushed to add healthy items and pass along nutritional information, for the most part the fast-food chains do things the way they want.

Most fast-food items contain no nutritional labeling and, further, do not reveal all their ingredients, even to the government. When they say "secret sauce," it's really a secret. They also have the big bucks to advertise extensively and very effectively.

A large chocolate malt, double burger with cheese and regular-sized french fries has on average 1,947 calories, mostly from fat. If you normally consume 2,000 calories a day, well, pass the water, because you've just about reached your limit.

DAY 6

Further, you've obtained hardly any of the vitamins and minerals you need and more than *twice* the amount of fat you should consume in a day. Considering that many people opt for the super-saving biggie sizes promoted so heavily, the fast-food remedy seems very close to being indictable for the nutritional rape of our nation.

WHAT YOU CAN DO

It is possible to eat a fast-food meal every once in a while. I make some recommendations for certain fast-food items, including Subway's six-inchers with under six grams of fat. My recommendations are among the few low-glycemic fast foods available. You can make fast food healthier if you make healthy choices, including salad bars, rice and veggie medleys, skim milk, and bean burritos. Watch the menus for items marked "healthy" and "low in fat," but if they can't produce *all* the nutritional info, assume there is a lack of nutrition in the product.

EATING HEALTHY, EATING OUT

Far better than fast foods are sit-down restaurants. However, the same rules apply: don't take their menu items at face value. Many times healthy-sounding foods come deep fried and drowning under a high-cream, buttery sauce or gravy.

Request meats to be grilled, not fried, and ask for sauces to be left off or served on the side. Seek out items from our low-glycemic list. You can nearly always request your vegetables steamed, and ask that meals are prepared as low in fat as possible.

Most restaurants accommodate substitutions in their menus. Exercise your right for healthy nutrition by asking for those substitutions. Steer clear of buffet lines—you'll always eat too much. Also, don't let them even tell you the specials—you're already special and don't need the temptation. You know how to eat healthy.

We all love to eat out, so do your body a favor and have it your way!

TAKE THIS THOUGHT TO BED WITH YOU

You need balance in everything—in work; in play; in physical, mental, and spiritual pursuits; in the friends you choose; and in the foods you eat.

Variety and balance are what keep life interesting. Life, even with sticking to all the healthy choices, can still be varied and interesting. Keep it fun, and you'll keep it up.

Day 6 has been wonderful, hasn't it? Sleep well!

Do it! Write it! Be it!

WHAT YOU ATE (If you swallowed it, write it down)

Breakfast: Lunch: Supper:

_____   _____   _____

_____   _____   _____

_____   _____   _____

_____   _____   _____

_____   _____   _____

_____   _____   _____

_____   _____   _____

_____   _____   _____

Snacks:

WHAT YOU DID

Cardiovascular Exercise   Time   Notes

_____   _____   _____

_____   _____   _____

_____   _____   _____

_____   _____   _____

What You Stretched and Moved

_____

_____

_____

_____

_____

_____

_____

SUCCESS LOG

WHAT YOU THOUGHT

_____
_____
_____
_____
_____
_____
_____
_____
_____
_____
_____
_____
_____
_____
_____
_____
_____
_____
_____
_____
_____
_____
_____
_____

ONLY 22 DAYS TO GO!

DAY 7

BRAIN POWER

It took six days for God to make earth and the heavens; on the seventh day He rested.

Regardless of your religion, rest is darn good advice because it is as important to good health as exercise. Put it to use today. Try some light stretching or perhaps some meditating this morning to limber up your body and mind.

EATING RIGHT

Today is a day of reflection. Eat healthy and make certain you get each of your macronutrients: fist-sized portions of protein and carbohydrates. Remember, the fat just comes along!

BREAKFAST

Breakfast on the go: Reach for your favorite meal replacement bar or smoothie. Add a piece of fresh fruit for an early morning snack and drink plenty of water.

Sit-down breakfast: Increase your protein for some good brain food and start out with a three-egg (or egg substitute) breakfast at home. Or, take yourself out to breakfast and order scrambled egg whites, eggs, or egg substitute with grilled onions and bell peppers, a side of cottage cheese, and a piece of whole-wheat toast with an all-fruit, no-sugar spread. Be sure to drink a glass of water with your meal.

LUNCH

Lunch on the go: Grab a deli salad without the bread and with a fist-sized portion of lean meat, some lettuce, tomato, avocado, and a little oil and vinegar. Have a breadstick and all the water you like.

Sit-down lunch: Make a sandwich with two slices of sourdough or whole-grain bread, a lean meat or grilled eggplant patty, a dab of low-fat mayonnaise, a slice of avocado, some lettuce or sprouts, and a slice of tomato. Drink all the water you want!

SUPPER

Supper on the go: Have a meal replacement shake, homemade, with extra protein, extra fresh fruit, and granola crunched up in the blender. Drink with a big glass of water.

Sit-down supper: Indulge yourself a little. Choose generous fist-sized portions of lean meat or a protein source, vegetables, and a carbohydrate. Finish with a medley of fresh berries in nonfat Cool Whip.

For a snack, have two big celery stalks stuffed with peanut butter, or a couple of slices of apple or cantaloupe with frozen nonfat vanilla yogurt, preferably plain.

Drink all the water or low-calorie water drinks you like!

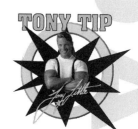

WORKOUT

Rest up today. Take care of yourself, your family, and your friends.

You're off the hook today, as far as resistance exercise is concerned.

For most muscles to respond to exercise, first they need work, then they need rest to grow and recuperate. Rest is important in exercise, and in life. A well-rested body (six to eight hours of sleep) generally has a much better immune system and a more alert attitude during the day.

Never underestimate the power of rest!

Instead of resistance exercise, why not participate in a little mental exercise with a review of Anatomy 101? Hide the answers on the right and see how many of these muscle groups you know:

DELTOIDS	the shoulders
TRAPEZIUS	the top of the shoulders, next to your neck
BICEPS	the front of the upper arm

TRICEPS	the back of the upper arm
FOREARMS	oh, come on!
PECTORALS	the muscles of the chest
ABDOMINALS or ABS	which you'll soon call abdominables!
OBLIQUES	the sides of your torso
GLUTEALS or GLUTES	your buttocks
QUADS or QUADRICEPS	your front thigh muscles
HAMSTRINGS	your rear upper leg muscles

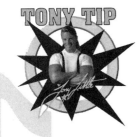

TONY TIP

Pamper yourself today. Get a massage or pedicure, go in the hot tub or take a long bath, or just curl up in a chair with your favorite paperback. Indulge yourself. Take yourself shopping. Maybe buy a new workout outfit, new tennis sneakers, or shorts.

It's good to be good to yourself.

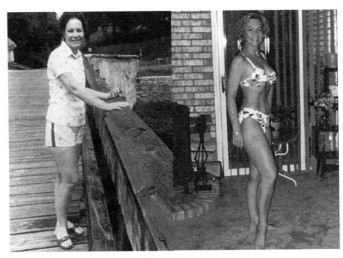

It's how the clothes fit, not what the scale hits. Fran deSorey from Rhode Island went from a size ten to a size five! She looks dynamite!

THE 40-40-20 AND 50-30-20 PLANS

Just because they eat every day, most people think they know about food. They know about taste, but I've discovered many people don't know diddly-squat about the nutritional value of their food.

Food is fuel for your body. Like a car, your body won't go without fuel, and the higher the grade of fuel, the better the performance.

The nutrients our bodies need are of three types:

▶ Macronutrients, which include carbohydrates, proteins, and fats, are those that are present in the body and are needed in large amounts.
▶ Micronutrients—vitamins, minerals, and other trace substances—are present in much smaller amounts.
▶ Water, though not usually thought of as a nutrient, is the third component that the body needs and is essential to life.

Each nutrient has specific functions, even though each nutrient interacts with others to carry out its functions.

In a nutshell, the macronutrients provide energy and help maintain and repair the body. Vitamins regulate the chemical processes that take place in the body. Minerals assist with this, and play a role in body maintenance as well, including the formation of new tissue, bones, teeth, and blood. Water provides a fluid medium necessary as a catalyst for all chemical reactions in the body, and also for the circulation of blood and removal of waste.

Your body is always burning a mixture of macronutrients for fuel to go about your daily tasks. The choice of all your nutrients becomes more critical when you

▶ try to limit the amount you eat in order to keep your bodyweight down, or
▶ ask a little more from your body, either in the form of workouts, sports or stress.

Both of these conditions apply to you right now, so read on!

A 40-40-20 diet is reasonable. It means from your total daily calories you should be deriving

▶ 40% in the form of protein
▶ 40% in the form of carbohydrates
▶ 20% in the form of fat

For most of you on this program and those who may wish to cut calories more drastically for weight loss, the best plan is

- 50% in the form of protein
- 30% in the form of carbohydrates
- 20% in the form of fat

Both these mixes will keep you from suffering the yo-yo syndrome whereby you lose weight, only to gain it all back—and more! You need balance in everything—especially your macronutrients!

Protein helps slow the burning of fuels and prevent spikes in your insulin levels. Insulin spikes are what lead to binge eating and unhealthy snacking. Protein also encourages lean muscle mass so that you will look your best from the exercise you perform.

CARBOHYDRATES AND FAT

At rest and at low levels of activity, carbohydrates provide 40% to 50% of the body's energy needs. Carbohydrates are the most efficient fuel for the body to use because they can be broken down to produce energy quickly. However, like fat, carbohydrates come in good and bad varieties. A good rule of thumb is to avoid simple sugars, corn syrup, fructose, and glycerin.

Fat—either from food or from body fat stores—also provides energy, but not as readily as carbohydrates. As a rule of thumb, avoid saturated fats such as the fat in red meat (always choose lean red meats) and corn oil. Polyunsaturated and monounsaturated fats such as the fat in most fish and olive oils are healthy to consume.

While all macronutrients are used for fuel, when they are eaten in excess of your caloric output, they are stored as fat! Therefore, you can't eat all the fat-free foods you want because even though you are not consuming fat, you are consuming carbohydrates. As with fat and protein, carbohydrates consumed in excess of your energy needs are stored as fat!

When counting calories, remember that carbohydrates and protein both contain four calories per gram. A gram of fat, however, produces more than twice, with nine calories.

A HEALTHY NUTRITION PLAN

A healthy diet—meaning one that is nutritious and also allows you to maintain your ideal bodyweight—isn't difficult to achieve once you learn to choose foods and nutrients that offer the best balance of nutrients for your body's needs.

Due to Americans' penchant toward overprocessing foods, our diet does not adequately provide the nutrition we need. For this reason, we have supplements.

Which vitamins and minerals are best? That answer is simple: a balance of them all. Vitamins and minerals work as teams in our bodies. As a matter of fact, without minerals, vitamins have no purpose. While our body can function, although poorly, with an inadequate supply of vitamins, we cannot survive without nature's essential minerals, no matter how small the mineral presence in our system may be.

Most Americans, men and women, need supplemental calcium. Antioxidants are also very important vitamins for everyone. Further, adequate protein—without the bad cholesterol of red meats—is essential and can easily be supplied by tasty, powder-based, protein-enriched shakes. These are all staples in my supplement cabinet.

TAKE THIS THOUGHT TO BED WITH YOU

A healthy choice every day keeps the doctor away.

Today is a day of reflection. Think about what you've accomplished by simply making it to Day 7.

If you need some inspiration to keep going, think about this:

- You've finally begun to change your eating habits and replace unhealthy choices with very healthy choices.
- You've learned a lot about what your body needs and what can improve your health.
- You've gained some extra energy.
- You're feeling the joy of accomplishment and of meeting a goal you've set.
- You may even have already lost a pound or two.
- You're feeling more rested, more content.
- Your kitchen reflects your commitment to this program.
- You're a winner!

Day 7 has been a good day, hasn't it? Be sure to write down what you've eaten, what you've done, and what you've thought about today.

Congratulations and sleep soundly. Dream big dreams, because you'll begin to realize them tomorrow! Visualize your dreams, and they will materialize!

Do it! Write it! Be it!

WHAT YOU ATE (If you swallowed it, write it down)

Breakfast: Lunch: Supper:

_____   _____   _____

_____   _____   _____

_____   _____   _____

_____   _____   _____

_____   _____   _____

_____   _____   _____

_____   _____   _____

Snacks:

WHAT YOU DID

Cardiovascular Exercise   Time   Notes

_____   _____   _____

_____   _____   _____

_____   _____   _____

Other Exercise   Time   Notes

_____   _____   _____

_____   _____   _____

_____   _____   _____

How You Rested

_____

_____

_____

_____

WHAT YOU THOUGHT

_____
_____
_____
_____
_____
_____
_____
_____
_____
_____
_____
_____
_____
_____
_____
_____
_____
_____
_____
_____
_____
_____
_____
_____
_____
_____

ONLY 21 DAYS TO GO!

WEEK 2:

Feeling Better, Looking Better

3

> While nutritionists argue endlessly over how we should eat for maximum health, the benefits of sensible exercise have never been questioned. Exercise is the single best thing you can do for your body, health, and longevity. All exercise relieves stress and can lower high blood pressure, increase energy levels, and improve the functioning of many of our most important organs, including the heart.

I've known many, many people who have exercised smart and consistently, and though most are now in their fifties, sixties, and seventies, I can say that each and every one looks, acts, and feels younger than their chronological age. That may be the best proof you need to incorporate a form of exercise into your daily routine, right now!

DAY 8

BRAIN POWER

Why is it that a lion's share of Americans vow to get in shape on New Year's Eve, then inevitably fail?

Because most people pick dreams and wishes as their resolutions—things like "lose weight" or "get in shape." These are not clear and definable goals. What you need in setting out on your path to accomplishment is to set specific goals and make the decision to carry them out. Check out the following:

- ▶ "At the end of this week I will feel stronger and better and will have learned how to harness my body's energy." That's a good one.
- ▶ "At the end of this week I will have made at least one positive change in my eating habits." Yes!
- ▶ "At the end of this week I will have established an eating and workout plan that will lead me to my ultimate goal of weight loss, better tone, improved self-image, and enhanced health."

Now those are the types of resolutions I want you to make! And, don't wait until New Year's. Start today.

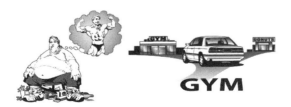

A wish changes nothing. A decision changes everything.
Illustration by Matt Gouig

EATING RIGHT

You're making the connection now! Seek out a healthy combination of protein, carbohydrates and fat. Select foods whenever possible from our chart on low-glycemic carbohydrates. Eat fist-sized servings. Keep your snacks healthy and natural.

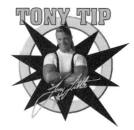

If you've been a soda lover all your life, try drinking the carbohydrateonated waters available in a variety of fruit flavors instead. For the truly soda-hooked, try Hansen's; for the less soda-hooked, try San Pellegrino with lemon.

BREAKFAST

Breakfast on the go: Feeling short on time? A meal replacement shake, a piece of fruit, lots of water, and a good vitamin/mineral supplement will send you on your way!

Sit-down breakfast: A fist-sized portion of turkey or chicken sausage; applesauce, low-fat, low-sugar yogurt, preferably plain, or cottage cheese; a glass of nonfat milk; and a slice of rye bread with just a hint of butter on it. One cup of coffee or tea, no sugar, black, or with a low-fat cream substitute. Try to eat the fruit or bread before the meat, if possible. Then, water, water, water.

LUNCH

Lunch on the go: While you're on the go, slip into a deli and get a lean meat sandwich, no mayonnaise, just mustard and greens. Have it on rye or pumpernickel bread with a big bottle of water. Have half a meal replacement bar for a snack later on.

Sit-down lunch: Grill a fist-sized portion of lean ground beef or chicken and have this with chopped onion. Also have kidney beans or black beans, a small amount of rice, and one medium tomato. Add grated cheese, salsa, shredded lettuce, plus a dollop of fat-free sour cream, and serve over six low-fat corn tortilla chips for a quick tortilla salad.

Have dried, canned, or fresh apricots for dessert. Drink at least eight ounces of water.

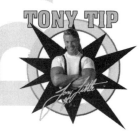

For a get-up-and-go snack, try some fresh or frozen berries in nonfat Cool Whip.

SUPPER

Supper on the go: It's time for a meal replacement drink or bar, or soup, followed by a piece of fresh fruit and plenty of water.

Sit-down supper: Have a fist-sized portion of chicken, fish, lean beef, or tofu with a fist-sized portion of beans, pasta, noodles, or rice. Take your pick from green peas, corn, green beans, raw carrots, or spinach. Enjoy trail mix with nuts and dried fruit for dessert.

Again, drink plenty of water. Water helps you lose body fat and it is great for your skin.

Healthy Nutrition and Fitness Is Simple

- Eat frequently
- Eat small portions
- Drink lots of water
- Increase activity

EXERCISE

In addition to our cardio and core training, which we will continue, we are going to add additional upper body, ab, and leg work.

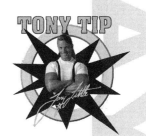

With resistance exercise, it is best to give the body at least a day's worth of recovery. That means you should never perform exactly the same exercise two days in a row, and many times it means you should put a day's rest between body parts.

CARDIOVASCULAR EXERCISE

We're doing 25 minutes of continuous cardio now. That's just enough to hit our fat-burning zone and plenty to ensure cardio conditioning for a healthy heart and stable sugar levels. One session is fine; two is divine.

Choices of exercises include marching around your living room, stationary cycling, walking outside, walking on a treadmill, gliding on the Gazelle Glider, or using the elliptical machine. Remember: keep movements fluid, energized, and brisk—not fast, just comfortable. If you feel you're breathing too hard, take the talk test: try to carry on a normal conversation for one minute without gasping for breath.

RESISTANCE EXERCISE

Ready, set, go. We're going to add some new moves to the old ones. So brace yourself to put out some energy today. We're going to do nine exercises.

What you put out is what makes the difference between those who succeed and those who fail. Remember, it's *now or never!* Come on, give new meaning to that old saying, "When the going gets tough, the tough get going!"

We're still going to stick to resistance exercise on three days a week. Ideally, that's on Monday, Wednesday, and Friday. If you miss a day, just pick up where you left off and keep on keeping on!

On the new exercises you'll only do one or two sets. Later in the week, I'll split these up. By the end of the week, your basic conditioning will be established and you'll be ready to tackle the higher loads for faster, more dramatic changes!

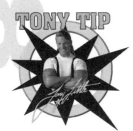

After a really great workout, pamper yourself. Treat yourself to a soothing soak in a hot tub. If you feel more sore than you'd like, a little Ibuprofen and light stretching throughout the day helps a lot.

P.S.: Pain that is so severe as to cause you discomfort is not good. If you push yourself too far, take a few days' rest and perform only the cardio before resuming the rest of your workout. This will not happen if you stick with the prescribed program, but for my overenthusiastic friends, pushing yourself too much too soon could make you very uncomfortable!

Get ready; this workout is the longest workout you'll perform. There's also a lot of muscle-learning, so let's get started!

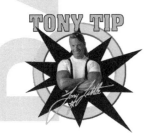

I cannot tell you how much to lift. You must determine that for yourself, and it will change from workout to workout. Find a weight that causes you to struggle just a bit for the last rep of your last set. That's how you determine a poundage that challenges and tones your muscles.

Just as your mood varies from day to day, you also have "strong days" and "weak days." Each day you need to adjust the effort you devote to your exercise. A cup of coffee or tea before your workout always helps to up the energy.

I can tell you that every time you exercise you need to squeeze the muscles being worked, and squeeze on the surrounding muscles that are supporting your movement. Squeeze everything you can!

1. Ab crunch (midsection):

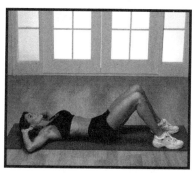 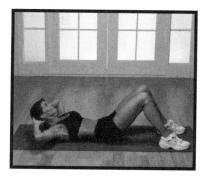

For at home or at the gym. Use 100% of your concentration to keep your entire body as tense as possible and to keep these movements slow and precise. Think squeeze and technique!

SET ONE: 10–15 repetitions
SET TWO: 10–15 repetitions

2. Reverse crunch (midsection):

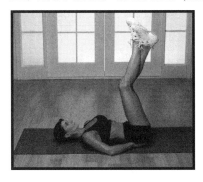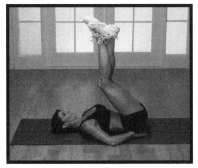

For at home or at the gym. Think technique! Don't let that lower back come too far off the ground, and breathe out as you bear down on the lower abs.

SET ONE: 10–15 repetitions
SET TWO: 10–15 repetitions

3. One-half squat (front and back of upper legs):

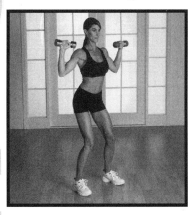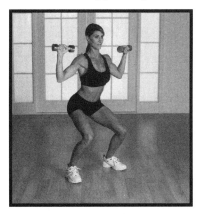

For at home or at the gym. Use your body weight or light, five- to 15-pound dumbbells. Today, try to go a bit deeper, until your upper legs are nearly parallel with the floor. Remember to *squeeze* and hold the weights as shown or lightly on the shoulders. Also go a bit slower; count to three on the way down and three on the way up! Squeeze on the way up.

SET ONE: 10–15 repetitions
SET TWO: 10–15 repetitions
SET THREE: 10–15 repetitions

4. Wide-stance squat (legs, inner thighs):

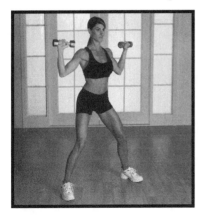 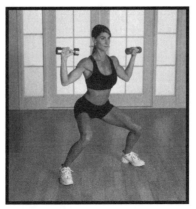

For at home or at the gym. Stand with your feet wider apart than shoulder width, toes pointed out at ten and two o'clock. If you are using weights, hold the weights (5- to 15-pound dumbbells) with elbows bent, palms facing forward. You can rest the ends of the dumbbells on your shoulders if more comfortable. Keep your back straight and eyes up, and squat down as far as comfortable. Then push back up with your legs. Perform this slowly. Count to four on the way down, and three on the way up, and *squeeze* your glutes!

SET ONE: 10–15 repetitions
SET TWO: 10–15 repetitions

4a. Leg press machine (quads, hamstrings, inner thighs):

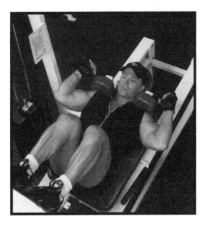 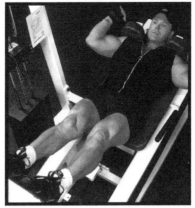

For the gym only. This versatile machine lets you focus on different parts of your upper leg musculature. To imitate the inner thigh work on the wide-stance squat, just place your feet out to the corners of the pads. If your feet are closer together, it better imitates the one-half squat. Begin by pushing the platform up past the slide guards. Be certain the weight is under your control at all times. Try one rep, and find a weight that is comfortable for 10 to 15 reps until you get used to the movement. The weight you choose should make you work hard to complete the last two reps. With abs, arms, and legs tense, lower the weight as far as comfortable and without stopping, reverse the motion and then push back to the top while squeezing your muscles.

SET ONE: 10–15 repetitions
SET TWO: 10–15 repetitions

5. Back row with chair (v-taper of back):

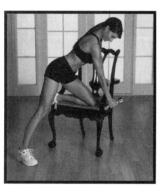 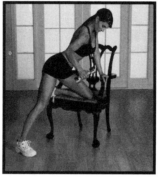 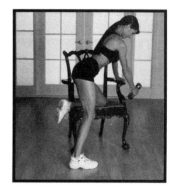

For at home or at the gym. This is a great exercise for strengthening the back. At home, find a sturdy armless chair and kneel on it as shown. In the gym, use a bench. Try and keep your chest almost parallel to the floor and your back straight. Balance on the chair with one arm and hold a dumbbell (use a light, 5- to 20-pound dumbbell) at arm's length in the other hand. Keeping your upper body tense, squeeze the dumbbell up to the side of your chest, elbows slightly bent out, then return to arm's length and stretch (but not the floor).

SET ONE: 10–15 repetitions
SET TWO: 10–15 repetitions

5a. Lat pulldown (back):

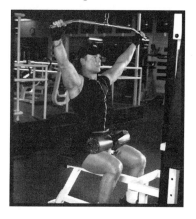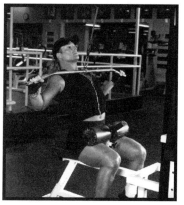

For the gym only. Any wide grip used in a pulling motion exercises the large muscles that run along the sides of the back. The lat pulldown is a classic that should be in everybody's gym routine. Use a weight heavy enough to make you really work for the last two reps. Position yourself so your thighs are secure under the pads. Reach up and take a wide grip (a little wider than shoulder width) on the bar. Squeeze your back muscles as you pull the bar down to your upper chest, arching slightly. Return, maintaining control.

> **SET ONE:** 10–15 repetitions
> **SET TWO:** 10–15 repetitions

6. Modified push-up or push-up (chest)

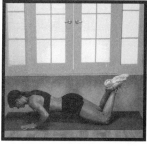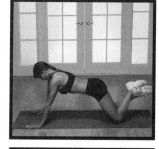

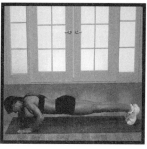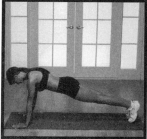

For at home or at the gym. You may perform this according to your conditioning. The easiest way is to perform it leaning against a table-high object. A more difficult push-up may be done lying flat on the floor and pushing up from your knees (as shown). The hardest form of push-up is lying flat on your stomach and pushing your entire body up from the floor while only your hands and toes are touching the floor. In all the different variations, your hands should be positioned just outside your shoulders, arms slightly bent out, elbows in line with your shoulders, back straight and your neck in a neutral position. Lower down to the point just before your chest touches the floor and then squeeze your chest muscles as you raise up, repeat.

SET ONE: 10–15 repetitions
SET TWO: 10–15 repetitions

6a. Chest press machine (chest):

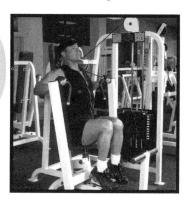 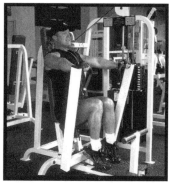

For the gym only. Adjust the seat on a chest press machine so that your hands are at chest level. Use a weight that makes the last two reps of each set hard to perform. With your feet firmly on the pad, tense your upper body, particularly your chest, and push the weight directly in front of you. Hold for one-half second at the peak contraction, return under control, and repeat. It's good to count one, two, three as you push out, and one and two on the return.

SET ONE: 10–15 repetitions
SET TWO: 10–15 repetitions

7. Shoulder press (shoulders):

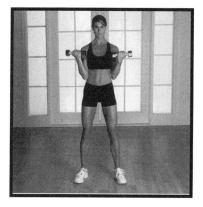
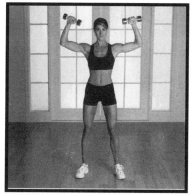

For at home or at the gym. This is a basic shoulder exercise. Stand with your feet shoulder-width apart, with your knees slightly bent. Holding a light, 5- to 15-pound dumbbell in each hand, bring them up to shoulder height, palms facing away from your body. In a slight arc, lift the dumbbells simultaneously above your head. Remember to *squeeze* and do not arch your back. Return them to the original position.

Avoid the tendency to arch your back and look up while performing this exercise. If you have trouble maintaining correct posture, you're probably using weights that are too heavy. In the gym you can use a special bench to support your back or use a shoulder press machine as discussed below.

SET ONE: 10–15 repetitions
SET TWO: 10–15 repetitions

7a. Seated shoulder press (shoulders):

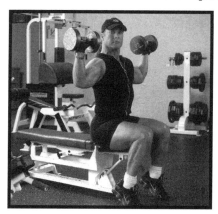
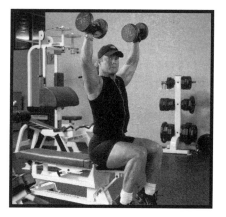

For the gym only. This version of the shoulder press allows you to use heavier dumbbells, about ten to 30 pounds. Sit on the end of a bench with the dumbbells in both hands. Begin with the dumbbells held as shown. Tensing your arms, shoulders, and torso, slowly bring the dumbbells up in an arc, as shown. Don't lock your arms out, and remember to squeeze. Return to the original position.

SET ONE: 10–15 repetitions
SET TWO: 10–15 repetitions

8. Triceps extension (back of upper arms):

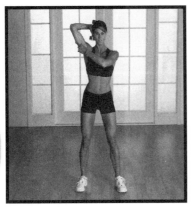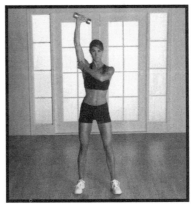

For at home or at the gym. Use your free arm to keep your upper arm stable during this movement. Begin with a light, 5- to 15-pound dumbbell held at arm's length. Keeping your upper arm in place, lower the weight as far as comfortable behind your head. Now bring the dumbbell back to arm's length as shown. Bring it back under control. Repeat for the other arm.

SET ONE: 10–12 repetitions
SET TWO: 10–12 repetitions

8a. Seated triceps pushdown on machine
(back of upper arms):

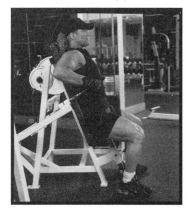
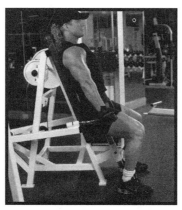

For the gym only. Sit in a triceps pushdown machine. In a warm-up set, start out light and find a weight that causes you to push hard. Grab both handles. Feet should be solid on the floor. Squeezing your triceps, press the handles down to arms' length without coming out of the seat. As you return the weight under control, keep tension on the triceps. Technique is very important. Return to the original position.

SET ONE: 10–12 repetitions
SET TWO: 10–12 repetitions

9. Dual bicep curl (biceps):

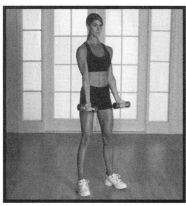
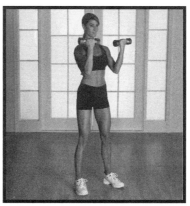

For at home or at the gym. Stand with your feet shoulder-width apart. For stability, you may want to lean your back against a wall. Begin with a 10- to 20-pound dumbbell in each hand, palms forward. *Squeeze* your biceps and abs as you curl the dumbbell up so that your palms are facing your shoulders. Slowly return with palms still facing out. This exercise may be performed with both dumbbells simultaneously, or by alternating one arm with the other.

SET ONE: 10–15 repetitions
SET TWO: 10–15 repetitions

9a. Barbell arm curl (biceps):

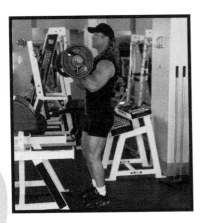 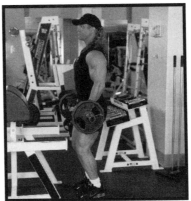

For the gym only. Stand in front of a rack and pick up a barbell in both hands. Use the heaviest barbell you can complete with eight to ten reps. Make certain your grip is centered on the bar, palms facing away from you. Squeeze your biceps and abs hard as you bring the weight up so your palms are facing your chest. Adjust weight for a squeezing technique that is fluid and controlled. Do not use overly heavy weights. Return slowly to the original position.

SET ONE: 10–15 repetitions
SET TWO: 10–15 repetitions

Whoa! Take a break! That was pretty darn good for your first week of a full-on resistance workout that exercises every major body part! I'm proud of you!

HEALTH SMARTS

FOUNTAIN OF YOUTH:
EXERCISE TO CREATE LIFELONG VITALITY AND HEALTH

The human body needs exercise to survive just as much as it needs food and water. You don't need to become a fitness freak or gym rat to do it. It can be done as simply as moving your body just a little bit more than you did yesterday.

How about practicing springing up from the couch and briskly walking about the house on your daily tasks? Bicycle riding is great, as are exercise tapes. So is a little yard work, or playing tag with your kids or walking your dog. How about dancing in your living room to your favorite music? Just about all leisure sports, such as golf, tennis, swimming, kayaking, skating, and cycling are all excellent forms of exercise.

That's all it takes to start, and a little exercise (as long as you progressively increase it) goes a long way in contributing to lifelong health.

Aerobic Exercise

Most of the forms of exercise mentioned above are aerobic in nature. In general, that means they are movements done in durations of 20 or more minutes. Done properly, they work up a sweat. To enable you to perform aerobic activities, your blood must deliver maximum oxygen to your muscles. This oxygenation improves with time, making your heart and entire cardiovascular system healthier.

Aerobic exercise is also a great fat-burner to keep your weight under control. If you are trying to lose weight, aerobic exercise is essential for accomplishing your goals. You'll have a healthier heart and lungs with aerobic exercise, as well as avoiding the health risks that come along with being overweight.

However, if you want to keep the vitality and strength of your youth for as long as you can, you need muscle too. And the indisputable champion of all time for building muscle is weight training!

Progressive Resistance: Weight Training

While aerobic exercise burns fat fast while you're performing it, progressive resistance exercise offers an important plus. Not only do you burn calories on the exercise floor, but you also burn calories when you leave it. It's a fact that weight training can increase your metabolism and keep you burning more calories for as long as 24 hours!

This metabolic increase also helps you to avoid the yo-yo syndrome of weight loss and weight gain. By toning and building the underlying muscle it helps to prevent age-related problems and injuries. Today, progressive resistance exercise has been accepted by all health authorities as the best means to improve health and body appearance.

For men, weight training will develop muscle rather quickly, but with my program you'll look more like Tom Cruise than Arnold Schwarzenegger. For women, today's programs will promote lean, toned, and curvaceous muscle that is more like a ballerina's than a discus thrower's.

In addition to producing attractive muscle tone, weight training will allow you to maintain (or build) muscle tissue that otherwise would naturally diminish with age. Weight-bearing exercise has also been proven effective in preventing and reversing osteoporosis. The loss of muscle and bone leaves the elderly weak and frail, susceptible to falls and broken bones, which makes weight training almost mandatory for people in their middle age.

Weight training also increases our metabolism by enhancing our body's muscle-to-fat ratio. One pound of muscle burns between 30 and 50 calories a day! Maintaining muscle mass will help you maintain a healthy bodyweight and is also a great way to keep you feeling vital and healthy.

We also lose growth hormone as we age. Diminished growth hormone plays a large role in decreased sex drive and energy. Weight training has been shown to have a beneficial effect on slowing growth hormone loss and may actually increase it.

TAKE THIS THOUGHT TO BED WITH YOU

Go to sleep knowing that you have embarked on a new path to great health and the best body you've ever dreamed of. Right now, you are doing the best thing you can possibly do for your body. You are exercising your right to a long, healthy, happy life.

You've done a lot. A whole lot. Relax, unwind, and I'll see you in the morning!

Do it! Write it! Be it!

WHAT YOU ATE (If you swallowed it, write it down)

Breakfast: Lunch: Supper:

_____   _____   _____

_____   _____   _____

_____   _____   _____

_____   _____   _____

_____   _____   _____

_____   _____   _____

Snacks:

WHAT YOU DID

Cardiovascular Exercise   Time   Notes

_____   _____   _____

_____   _____   _____

Resistance Exercise   Reps/Sets/Weight   Notes

_____   _____   _____

_____   _____   _____

_____   _____   _____

_____   _____   _____

_____   _____   _____

_____   _____   _____

_____   _____   _____

WHAT YOU THOUGHT

ONLY 20 DAYS TO GO!

DAY 9

BRAIN POWER

Hello and good morning, warrior! Jump out of bed today, stand with your feet together, and take one giant step with your right foot! Getting off on the right foot always starts the day in a better way.

And when you pass that mirror, check yourself out. Looking good? Standing taller? Feeling happier?

It's good to check your progress. Have you tried on a pair of tight pants to see if they're fitting better? Have you reviewed your logbooks to see how your attitude—and conditioning—have changed?

If you haven't, do it now!

EATING RIGHT

If you haven't already, stock up now on those prepared meal replacement drinks and/or bars along with a can of protein mix. (Remember to read the labels and look for protein content at about 19 to 23 grams and carbohydrates at about 6 to 10 grams a serving. Always look for a high-protein, low-carbohydrate combination.)

Also, beware of "hidden" carbohydrates. The two you'll most likely run into are maltodextrin and glycerin (glycerine, glycerol), which are used as fillers and technically are not carbohydrates. However, once absorbed in your body they convert and store themselves as fat, just like a high-glycemic carbohydrate. These are rarely listed as carbohydrates on the food label, so if you see them in the ingredient list be aware the product is packing more carbohydrate calories than the label shows!

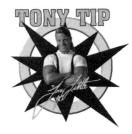

Reach for fresh fruit and vegetables when you need a snack. Add a slice of cheese, some low-fat yogurt, preferably plain, some cottage cheese, or a little peanut butter for protein and for a healthier between-meal snack.

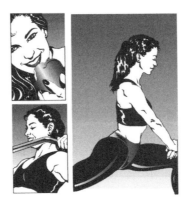

Eat right, exercise right, look right.
Illustration by Matt Gouig

BREAKFAST

Breakfast on the go: High-protein, low-carbohydrate meal replacement prepared drinks or bars are the quickest way to go. Be careful not to replace more than two meals per day. Try to find products that are loaded with extra vitamins and minerals to keep your diet balanced. Drink lots of water!

Sit-down breakfast: Mix a low-fat, low-sugar yogurt, preferably plain, with a few walnuts or almonds, and half a cup of strawberries, raspberries, blackberries, and/or blueberries. Add a tablespoon of vanilla protein powder. Enjoy with a morning cup of coffee, tea, apple juice, or nonfat milk.

Now step out with that right foot again and continue the day!

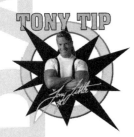

Always include a source of protein in your three major meals. This can come from a variety of vegetables and beans, dairy, or lean meat. Protein is king!

LUNCH

Lunch on the go: Have some low-fat, low-sugar yogurt, preferably plain, a piece of fruit, and a meal replacement bar.

Sit-down lunch: Have one fist-sized lean hamburger patty, turkey patty, or a low-fat veggie burger (like Boca) cooked on a George Foreman grill or fried with Pam. Flavor it lightly in A-1 sauce or ketchup. Serve with a third of an avocado, a cup of cottage cheese, and two slices of rye or pumpernickel bread.

Have an apple or two apricots for dessert. Drink at least eight ounces of water. Remember: water, water, water!

SUPPER

Supper on the go: Swing by a to-go salad bar (they have one at most big supermarkets) and load up on the fresh vegetables, tuna, hard-boiled eggs, or another protein-rich topping. Add just two tablespoons of your favorite dressing. Drink plenty of water and have half a meal replacement bar or shake for dessert.

Sit-down supper: Grill or bake your choice of flank steak, sole, or soy patties. Add a fist-sized portion of green beans, peas, cabbage, spinach, or corn, and a cup of macaroni, spaghetti, or fettuccine with a tablespoon of marinara sauce.

Drink lots of water and add a fresh fruit for dessert.

WORKOUT

Can you guess what's in store? I will be leading you for the next 19 days, but after that you'll be implementing this lifestyle on your own. So think about what you're doing! Learn as we go, and when we finish, you'll have a new and healthy habit.

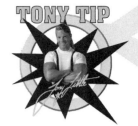

Don't let cardio be boring! Watch the second hand on the clock, and try turning up the energy/speed for just one minute, every four or five minutes. Challenge yourself. It's called interval training. Let's see if we can get a little teeth-gritting grimace outta you!

Better yet, let's see if we can get you to sweat!

Jack LaLanne, the father of fitness, once said, "To stay in optimum health all we need to do is sweat a little, every day." Jack is still in great shape today at 85!

CARDIOVASCULAR EXERCISE

Today it's 25 minutes of cardio (walking, marching, dancing, cycling, gliding, or stepping). Get goin'. You may want to check your resting heart rate as we up the ante on our cardio output.

Target Heart Rate

The simplest way to calculate your Target Heart Rate is to subtract your age from 220. This number is the maximum times a healthy heart should beat in one minute. If you are just beginning, your Target Heart Rate should be between 60% and 65% of your maximum heart rate. At the end of this program it should be 70% to 75%, and after two months you may be ready to raise it to the advanced rate of 80% to 85%.

TARGET HEART RATE RANGE
(Beats Per 10 Seconds)

Age	Beginner (50-60%)	Intermediate (60-70%)	Advanced (70-90%)
20-25	16-20	20-23	23-29
26-30	16-19	19-22	22-28
31-35	15-19	19-22	22-27
36-40	15-18	18-21	21-27
41-45	15-18	18-21	21-26
46-50	14-17	17-20	20-25
51-55	14-17	17-20	20-25
56-60	13-16	16-19	19-24
61-65	13-16	16-18	18-23
66-70	13-15	15-18	18-23

There are many other charts that determine your Target Heart Rate by factoring in age and conditioning level. Many of these are available on the Internet by searching for Target Heart Rate calculators.

During exercise, the easiest way to check your heart rate is to place the tips of your middle and index fingers in the groove of your throat just to the side of the Adam's apple. Count the heartbeats for ten seconds and multiply the number of beats by six. If you are not within your range, you may need to adjust your workout. After cooling down, check your pulse rate again. It should be below 100 before you stop moving.

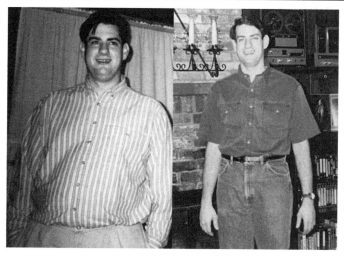

Consistency is key.
Carl Lander from Pennsylvania lost 75 pounds on Tony's programs.
Carl is a pro, he's kept the weight off!

Reminder: Don't forget to keep track of what you eat, do and think in your logbooks!

RESISTANCE EXERCISE

No resistance training today! Your body needs to rest. On this active rest day take a few minutes to do some stretches. Then come up with four ways to increase energy output while doing simple, mundane tasks—for example, walking faster, skipping, running up the stairs, vacuuming, doing yard work, or sweeping the floor in half your usual time. Be creative, and keep it movin'.

HEALTH SMARTS

THE I-CAN-DO-IT ATTITUDE!

If there is one undeniable fact about exercise, it is that no one ever got in shape just by thinking about it. You have got to do the action to reap the rewards. There are hundreds of terrific routines and approaches to exercise, and all of them have merit—that is, if you do them!

DAY 9

Sticking with an exercise program can be a tough problem for seasoned trainers as well as newcomers. Fortunately, there are a few practical tips to help keep you motivated and on your program:

1. Set short-term goals—a half-inch skinnier, a half-pound lighter, or even a half-size lower in clothes. A measuring tape, scale, and skin calipers are great for charting your progress. Keep track of your progress on a weekly basis—success is the best motivator of all.

2. Treat your workout not as a luxury, but as a necessity: like work and meals. Don't give yourself an option to back out. Put your workouts at a higher priority than errands, socializing, and other distractions.

3. Always be prepared. Have a separate area set aside in your home where you go to work out. If you work out at a gym, carry an extra set of gym clothes and shoes in your car or keep them at the office.

4. A little is better than none. When pressed for time or other commitments, shorten your workout rather than skipping it completely. If you choose this option, try to put a little more effort into every move you do.

5. Set a specific and consistent time for your workouts. Make certain this is a time that works with your schedule, then mark it on all your calendars.

6. After every workout, remind yourself how good you feel. Take a moment to applaud yourself for putting in the effort. Put a mental bookmark in your thoughts and recall how good you feel after a workout to help you stay on your program, for life.

TAKE THIS THOUGHT TO BED WITH YOU

Your first step in winning anything in life is to believe in yourself. Many are the times that I could have given up. There were days that I was physically and emotionally impaired and it hurt just to think about getting up and moving. But I believed I could get back on my feet. I believed I would be strong again. I believed I would not cause people to lower their eyes in pity at the sight of me.

I believed, because I'd already seen such a transformation in myself and others. It can be done. Millions have already proven it. There is no magic. Do the program, reap the rewards. But first, you must believe you can do it.

Day 9, outta here! Good night!

Do it! Write it! Be it!

WHAT YOU ATE (If you swallowed it, write it down)

Breakfast: Lunch: Supper:

_____   _____   _____
_____   _____   _____
_____   _____   _____
_____   _____   _____
_____   _____   _____
_____   _____   _____
_____   _____   _____

Snacks:

WHAT YOU DID

Cardiovascular Exercise   Time   Notes

_____   _____   _____
_____   _____   _____
_____   _____   _____
_____   _____   _____

Other Activities

_____
_____
_____
_____
_____
_____
_____

SUCCESS LOG

WHAT YOU THOUGHT

ONLY 19 DAYS TO GO!

DAY 10

BRAIN POWER

We're more than one-third of the way through and you're feelin' it, right? Sleeping a little more soundly, feeling a bit more empowered, getting in touch with your body—especially this week.

Physical fitness is about getting your body in shape, but it's not all physical. You need a mental mind-set as well. That mind-set reinforces your new love affair with fitness. That mind-set also needs to come into play every time you exercise.

Don't just *do* the move, *feel* the move. Use your brain to intensify it! Use your mind to force energy into your muscles. When you move it, *I want you to really move it!*

DID YOU KNOW . . . ?: Using your muscles is a bit like using your brain—you access only a small portion of its potential! If you were to take your muscles out of your body and place them on a rack, they could hold onto hundreds—sometimes thousands—of pounds.

Your strength gives out as a protective device to keep you from hurting your ligaments and tendons—or tearing a muscle. But that mechanism kicks in early—long before you're really in danger.

Learning to push that limit is important. And it can only come with mental power. We've all heard stories about regular people—in extreme situations such as needing to save a loved one—who have managed to perform incredible feats of strength.

You have the power. Use it.

EATING RIGHT

Is making healthy choices becoming easier? It should be. Be sure you are not denying yourself too many calories.

If you feel sluggish, take your temperature first thing in the morning. If your temperature falls below normal two days in a row, it's a sign that you are not eating enough calories and that you need to increase your portions in this meal plan.

BREAKFAST

Breakfast on the go: By now your fridge and cupboards should be full of easy meal replacements—prepared drinks, bars, soups, fresh vegetables, fruits, and low-fat dairy—to be used when you're on the go. Grab one, and go for it!

Sit-down breakfast: A bowl with a fist-sized portion of low-sugar, high-fiber cereal and low-fat milk. One cup of coffee or tea, no sugar, black or with a low-fat cream substitute, or apple juice.

LUNCH

Lunch on the go: A fist-sized portion of lean deli meat, a low-fat, low-sugar yogurt, preferably plain, and a piece of fruit. Drink plenty of water and munch on a handful of nutty trail mix for dessert.

Sit-down lunch: Mix up a great salad of two handfuls of cooked macaroni, plus diced broccoli, celery, red pepper, yellow pepper, green onion, and tomatoes. For the dressing, mix a tablespoon of white wine vinegar, two tablespoons seasoned rice vinegar, a teaspoon of olive oil, a pinch of garlic, a pinch of basil, a dash of salt, and a dash of black pepper. Top with Parmesan cheese.

Have an apple or orange for dessert. Drink at least eight ounces of water.

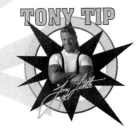

Don't forget to pick out healthy carbohydrate choices from the list of low-glycemic carbohydrates.

SUPPER

Supper on the go: Have a meal replacement drink or bar, a piece of fruit, and all the water you can drink.

Sit-down supper: Simple. Choose a fist-sized piece of lean meat or tofu, grilled. Now go to the list of low-glycemic carbohydrates and choose a fist-sized portion of vegetables (yellow, green, or red), a fist-sized portion of carbohydrates, and one piece of fruit.

Always drink plenty of water with your meals.

WORKOUT

Don't forget to stretch! Do this in the morning when you first wake up, or in the evening when you start to relax for bed. Or, combine stretching with your workouts. Work it into your routine somehow. Check out page 301 for more stretching tips.

CARDIOVASCULAR EXERCISE

Push it to 30 minutes today. That's right. You can do it!

Watch the clock. Pick one of your favorite forms of cardio: dancing, marching, riding a stationary bike, gliding, power walking, cycling, skipping, or following a video.

What are you waiting for? Get to it!

> ## You are what you eat.
> ## You are what you do.
> ## You are what you think.
>
> **W**rite everything down in the logbooks, and think about it!

RESISTANCE EXERCISE

Put some mental muscle into your workout today. Work a little harder. *Think* about the muscle you're working.

Ideally, you should have a mirror in your workout area. It helps to watch your muscles contract and relax.

Remember that PRE scale for cardio? Well, today I want you to work toward a resistance exercise PRE of 7 or 8 on a scale of 1 to 10. That means you need to struggle for those last reps, or increase the resistance!

Today's routine will work the large muscles of the back, chest, legs, and abs.

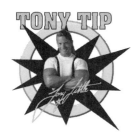
Cardio exercise works the fastest to help you burn calories and lose weight. Resistance training takes longer, but its effects are greater because it builds lean muscle mass, which in turn increases your metabolism to burn more calories throughout the day—even while at rest!

1. Ab crunch (midsection):

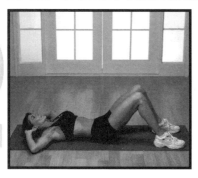 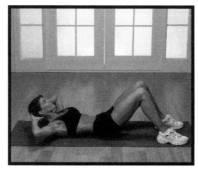

For at home or at the gym. Keep your body as tense as possible and keep these movements slow and precise. Think *squeeze* and technique!

> **SET ONE:** 10–15 repetitions
> **SET TWO:** 10–15 repetitions
> **SET THREE:** 10–12 repetitions

2. Reverse crunch (midsection):

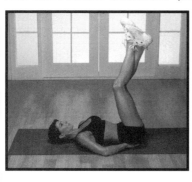 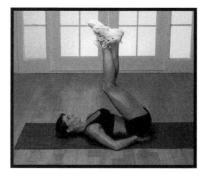

For at home or at the gym. Think technique! Don't let that lower back come too far off the ground, and breathe out as you bear down on the lower abs.

SET ONE: 10–15 repetitions
SET TWO: 10–15 repetitions
SET THREE: 10–12 repetitions

3. Lying back extension (lower back):

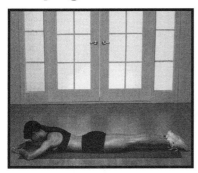 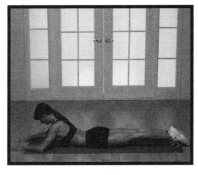

For at home or at the gym. Keep your neck in a neutral position. Allow your back to stretch as well as flex, and don't forget to squeeze. This will help keep you from getting lower back pain.

SET ONE: 10–15 repetitions
SET TWO: 10–15 repetitions

4. One-half squat (quadriceps, gluteals, hamstrings):

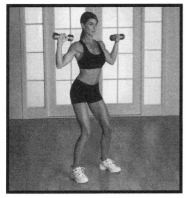 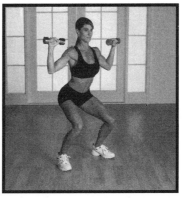

For at home or at the gym. Use bodyweight or light, 5- to 10-pound dumbbells. Today try to go deeper—maybe halfway down. Never bottom out where your upper legs hit your lower legs. Also, go a bit slower; count to three on the way down and squeeze and count to three on the way up!

SET ONE: 10–15 repetitions
SET TWO: 10–15 repetitions
SET THREE: 10–15 repetitions

5. Stationary lunge (front and back of upper legs and buttocks):

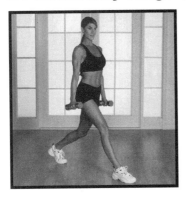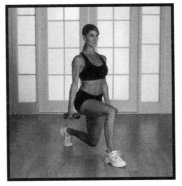

For at home and at the gym. Use only your bodyweight or light, five- to ten-pound dumbbells. Perform this lunge by standing upright and taking a large stride forward with your right leg. This is the start position. Bending your right knee, let your left knee trail as low as comfortable, but do not touch the floor. Keep your forward knee over the ball of your foot. If it extends too far, your stride is too short. If it doesn't go over the ball of your foot, your stride is too long. Stand back up to the start position—think *squeeze*. You should feel it the most in your front leg. Concentrate on that front leg pushing you back up. Finish all your reps for one leg before moving to the other leg.

SET ONE: 8–10 repetitions per leg
SET TWO: 8–10 repetitions per leg

5a. Leg extension (front upper legs):

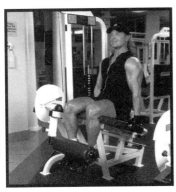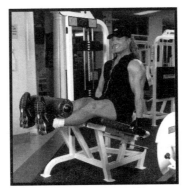

For at the gym only. Position yourself in a leg extension machine so the front of your ankles are secure behind the pads. Hold onto the side handles. Squeeze your quads as you extend your legs straight out in front, and keep your toes pointed back to you. Tighten your abs. Keep your buttocks from coming up off the seat. Hold for one second at the peak contraction, then lower the bar. In addition to the seated version shown, standing and prone versions of the hamstring machine are popular. Adjust the weight so it is not too heavy, but comfortable to perform a set.

SET ONE: 10–15 repetitions
SET TWO: 10–15 repetitions

6. Back Row with chair (v-taper of back):

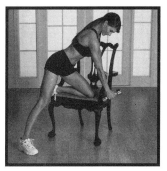 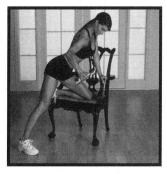 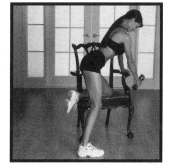

For at home or at the gym. This is a great exercise for strengthening the back. At home, find a sturdy armless chair and kneel on it as shown. In the gym, use a bench. Try and keep your chest almost parallel to the floor and your back straight, balance on the chair with one arm and hold a dumbbell (use a light, 5- to 20-pound dumbbell) at arm's length in the other hand. Keeping your upper body tense, squeeze the dumbbell up to the side of your chest, elbow slightly bent out, then return to arm's length and stretch (but not to the floor).

SET ONE: 10-15 repetitions
SET TWO: 10-15 repetitions

6a. Back row machine (back):

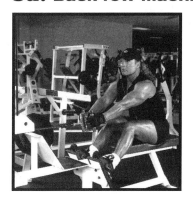 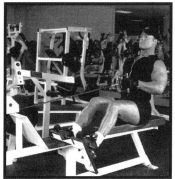

For the gym only. If you have access to the gym, perform this after performing the side deltoid throw. Grab the close-grip handles on a rowing machine with a 45-degree back, then push back with your legs until there is tension on the cable. Do not lean backwards; keep your back straight. From this position, pull the handles close to your body and squeeze your shoulder blades at the peak of the movement. Return, and stretch. Adjust the weight so 10 reps would be comfortable, but 15 is a little harder.

SET ONE: 10–15 repetitions
SET TWO: 10–15 repetitions

7. Modified push-up or push-up (chest):

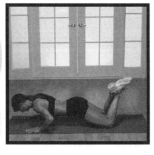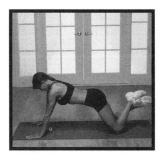

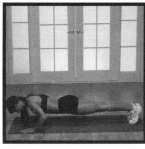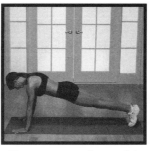

For at home or at the gym. You may perform this according to your conditioning. The easiest way is to perform it leaning against a table-high object. A more difficult push-up may be done lying flat on the floor and pushing up from your knees (as shown). The hardest form of push-up is lying flat on your stomach and pushing your entire body up from the floor while only your hands and toes are touching the floor. In all the different variations, your hands should be positioned just outside your shoulders, arms slightly bent out, elbows in line with your shoulders, back straight and your neck in a neutral position. Lower down to the point just before your chest touches the floor and then squeeze your chest muscles as you raise up, repeat.

SET ONE: 10–15 repetitions
SET TWO: 10–15 repetitions
SET THREE: 10–15 repetitions

7a. Chest press machine (chest):

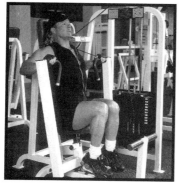 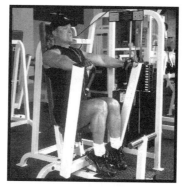

For the gym only. With your feet firmly on the pad, tense your upper body, particularly your chest, and push the weight directly in front of you. Hold for one-half second at the peak contraction and *squeeze*, then return to the original position under control. Adjust weight by testing one rep. Make sure it is comfortable for you to do a set to start, and then gradually challenge yourself to more.

> **SET ONE:** 10–15 repetitions
> **SET TWO:** 10–15 repetitions
> **SET THREE:** 10–15 repetitions

8. Shoulder press (shoulders):

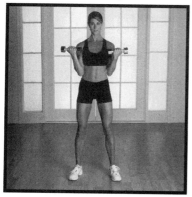 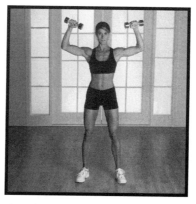

For at home or at the gym. This is a basic shoulder exercise. Stand with your feet shoulder-width apart, with your knees slightly bent. Holding a light, 5- to 15-pound dumbbell in each hand, bring them up to shoulder height, palms facing away from your body. In a slight arc, lift the dumbbells simultaneously above your head. Return to the original position.

> **SET ONE:** 10–15 repetitions
> **SET TWO:** 10–15 repetitions

8a. Seated shoulder press (shoulders):

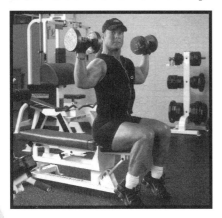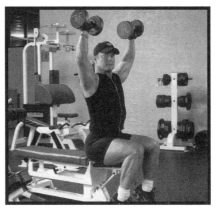

For the gym only. Begin with eight- to 20-pound dumbbells held as shown. Tensing your arms, shoulders, and abs, slowly bring the dumbbells up in an arc (as shown). Keep your palms facing forward. Return to the original position.

> **SET ONE:** 10–15 repetitions
> **SET TWO:** 10–15 repetitions

9. Triceps extension (back of upper arms):

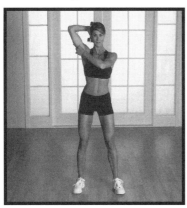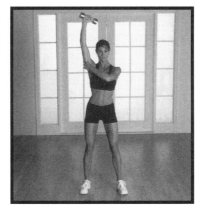

For at home or at the gym. Use your free arm to keep your upper arm stable during this movement. Begin with one light, 5- to 15-pound dumbbell held at arm's length. Keeping your upper arm in place, lower the dumbbell behind your head. Squeeze back up. Repeat for the other arm.

> **SET ONE:** 10–12 repetitions
> **SET TWO:** 10–12 repetitions

9a. Seated triceps pushdown on machine (back of upper arms):

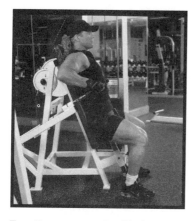 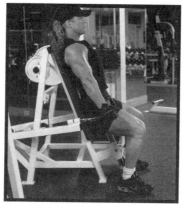

For the gym only. Sit in a triceps pushdown machine and grab both handles. Feet should be solid on the floor. Squeezing your triceps, press the handles down to arms' length. Return to the original position. Adjust weight and check with one rep. Find weight that you can squeeze down for one set. Concentrate on technique.

SET ONE: 10–12 repetitions
SET TWO: 10–12 repetitions

10. Dual bicep curl (biceps):

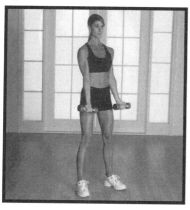 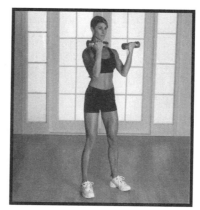

For at home or at the gym. Begin with a medium-weight, 10- to 30-pound dumbbell in each hand, palms forward. *Squeeze* your biceps and abs as you curl the dumbbell up so that your palms are facing your shoulders. Return slowly with your palms facing forward.

SET ONE: 10–15 repetitions
SET TWO: 10–15 repetitions

10a. Barbell arm curl (biceps):

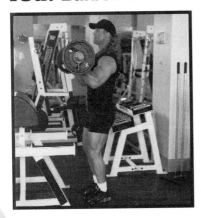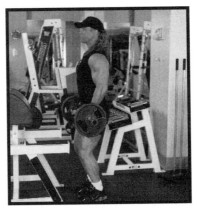

For the gym only. Stand in front of a rack and pick up a barbell in both hands. Use a medium-weight, 24- to 45-pound barbell. Make certain your grip is centered, palms facing away from you. Squeeze your biceps hard as you bring the weight up so your palms are facing your chest. Return slowly. Adjust weight for a squeezing technique that is fluid and controlled.

SET ONE: 10–15 repetitions
SET TWO: 10–15 repetitions

Finish off with some light stretching, especially for those hamstrings in the back of your legs. Remember, never force a stretch, or bounce. Slow and easy is your motto.

HEALTH SMARTS

LARGE MUSCLES BURN MORE CALORIES—WORK 'EM!

I have nothing against exercising the wrists, forearms, and ankles, but I would not devote much time to them. Many of these small muscle groups benefit when you are working the major groups anyway. What I do care about are the major muscle groups in your body: the chest, back, and legs.

These muscle groups are large and burn the most calories while you work them. They also work faster at raising your body's ratio of lean muscle mass in order to increase your metabolism and keep the weight off. Therefore, your resistance routine concentrates on those big muscle groups.

You Can't Spot Reduce

Everyone wants a smaller waistline. Therefore many people only train their abs. That's fine, and satisfying, but it is not the quickest way to get that torso centerpiece in shape. Working the larger muscles and burning more calories is a far quicker way to lose the total body fat that is covering your abs.

A lot of people say to me, "Tony, how do I get abs?" I have to laugh when I tell them, "Everyone has abs. If you didn't, you would look more like a rubber chicken. Abs stand you up, sit you down, and hold you upright when you walk." The truth is that everyone has abs, they just have too much fat covering them up so no one can see them!

Many women hold the majority of their weight in their hips, buttocks, and thighs. This is referred to as the pear shape. Feminine genetics cause women to store extra fat on the hips and buttocks. In certain cases, this can lead to very disproportionate dimensions that look almost as if two different bodies were joined at the waist! This is one good reason women should not eat the high-glycemic carbohydrates—those are the ones most likely to be stored in the hip and thigh area!

It has been shown in several studies that extra work on the large muscles of the lower body reduces its overall size. That's why this routine has you doing a lot of leg work. Even if you're from a long line of pear-shaped people, this program can actually fight those genetics. Fighting genetics isn't easy—and neither are your workouts as we progress—but in most cases exercise can reshape the body in spite of its programming.

Whether you are one of those women fighting lower-body bulges, or just a person who wants to lose weight, shape up, strengthen up, and look your best, the extra emphasis on the legs in this program will go a long way to accomplish your goals.

Do the Work; Reap the Rewards

The legs are composed of large, hardworking muscles and it takes a lot of energy to give them the workout they need. This is why many people shy away from these energy-burning core movements, and opt instead to use the leg extension or abductor/adductor machines. These machines have their purpose but they can't match the intensity and compound nature of a lunge, squat, or push-up.

Don't shy away from these exercises that are included in all your workouts. Do them with energy, gusto, and verve. They will pay off with faster results and a more lean, beautiful you!

Whatever you can conceive, and believe, you will achieve.

Say this to yourself 20 times tonight: *conceive, believe, achieve.*

You have the power. You will do it. You can do it!

God bless you, and good night.

DAY 10

Do it! Write it! Be it!

WHAT YOU ATE (If you swallowed it, write it down)

Breakfast: Lunch: Supper:

_____   _____   _____

_____   _____   _____

_____   _____   _____

_____   _____   _____

_____   _____   _____

_____   _____   _____

_____   _____   _____

Snacks:

WHAT YOU DID

Cardiovascular Exercise   Time   Notes

_____   _____   _____

_____   _____   _____

Resistance Exercise   Reps/Sets/Weight   Notes

_____   _____   _____

_____   _____   _____

_____   _____   _____

_____   _____   _____

_____   _____   _____

_____   _____   _____

DAY 10 ⬇

SUCCESS LOG

WHAT YOU THOUGHT

_____
_____
_____
_____
_____
_____
_____
_____
_____
_____
_____
_____
_____
_____
_____
_____
_____
_____
_____
_____
_____
_____
_____
_____
_____
_____
_____
_____
_____

ONLY 18 DAYS TO GO!

DAY 11

BRAIN POWER

Each morning we wake to a new day. Whether it's sunny or gray, the birds wake to morning with a song. Do the same.

Music motivates us to move. Think upbeat. Think with a beat. Snap your fingers. Tap your feet. Get movin'. Stay movin'.

> **H**ow many summers do you have left? Make the most of all of them. Who knows how many more summers you might have now that you've begun taking better care of yourself!

EATING RIGHT

Eating well is about making healthy choices. The adjustments you've made in your meals thus far are just beginning to have an effect on your body.

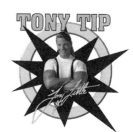

Keep it simple. You are what you eat. Eat too much fat, and you'll be much too fat.

Four simple rules will help you lose weight:

- *Eat frequently*
- *Eat small, fist-sized portions*
- *Drink lots and lots of water*
- *Increase your activity*

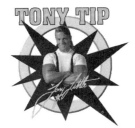

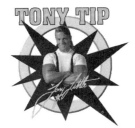

Keep hard-boiled eggs and lean deli meat handy for quick, high-protein between-meal snacks!

BREAKFAST

Breakfast on the go: High-protein, low-carbohydrate prepared drinks or bars may be used to replace one or two meals a day. Try to balance them out with a piece of fruit either with breakfast, or as a snack an hour later. Drink plenty of water, water, water!

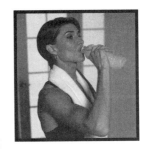

Sit-down breakfast: In a teaspoon of olive oil in a Pam-sprayed pan, scramble egg substitute or mix tofu with broccoli, red peppers, green peppers, onion, and zucchini. Put into a warm corn tortilla. Add salsa to taste (the thermogenic properties of salsa help burn calories). Have one cup of coffee or tea, no sugar, black or with a low-fat cream substitute and all the water you can drink.

LUNCH

Lunch on the go: While I don't recommend fast food, it's okay according to the Glycemic Index to dive into a local Taco Bell for two plain bean burritos with extra lettuce and cheese. Or try the soft chicken tacos. Drink lots and lots of water!

Sit-down lunch: Brown a portion of lean ground turkey or beef with onions and bell pepper. Add prepared pasta sauce and spoon over two handfuls of your favorite cooked pasta. Enjoy with steamed broccoli and fruit for dessert. Drink at least eight ounces of water.

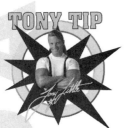

Throw away your scale (or at least hide it). The scale can be your enemy. A tight-fitting skirt or pair of shorts or pants is your best measurement of your progress. Your proportions will change before the number on the scale does.

SUPPER

Supper on the go: Grab a meal replacement shake or smoothie. Make it yourself with fresh fruit and additional low-fat yogurt, preferably plain and/or extra protein. Drink lots of water.

Sit-down supper: Have you had your fish today? Try a salmon steak, mahi-mahi, sole, or swordfish, fist-sized, broiled in the oven or on a George Forman grill. Add a cup of wild rice and a medley of mixed green, orange, and yellow vegetables (broccoli, carrots, yellow peppers) with mushrooms, lightly stir-fried in a tablespoon of olive oil.

Always drink plenty of water with your meals. A diet soda is in order tonight if you prefer.

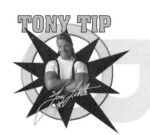

Fad diets don't work for long. Make a vow to yourself to never diet again. You need a lifestyle plan for healthy eating. You need to make healthy choices a habit. You're almost halfway there!

WORKOUT

Another 30 minutes of cardio. Today you'll be using the interval method by varying your speed and effort. Studies have shown that using the interval technique during cardio burns more calories than training harder at a consistent pace.

Plus, it makes it more exciting! If you're having trouble getting so much cardio time in, split it up with half in the morning and half in the evening. And use my Cardio Two-Minute Warning: spend the last two minutes of every cardio workout going as fast and hard as you can, then cool down for five minutes. We'll also be working the shoulders, arms, abs, and legs today.

CARDIOVASCULAR EXERCISE

Pick your form of cardio: walking, marching, stair climbing, gliding, going on the treadmill, cycling, or dancing. Whatever form you choose, watch the clock, and at five-minute intervals increase your intensity. Strive for one minute at high speed, but if all you can do is 15, 30, or 45 seconds, that's fine too. Your body adjusts very quickly to regular cardio and you'll be increasing that time in just days!

How to Succeed at Exercise

- Concentrate on tensing (squeezing) your muscles—even those that aren't working
- Think technique; get the most out of every rep
- Increase resistance and range of motion
- Be consistent and keep a log

Don't forget to record what you eat, what you do, and what you think.

RESISTANCE EXERCISE

Once again, today is your rest day. Stay active though, and seek out calorie-burning things to do. Ever notice that most busy people are thin people? It's true, and it can be true for you!

Even though you are resting, your abdominals can always use some extra work. Your abs are your center of power. Almost everything you do requires the abs to help stabilize you. For this reason and in contrast to some other muscles, the abs like to be worked a lot, and often. Let's add a new ab move today.

1. Compound crunch (abdominals):

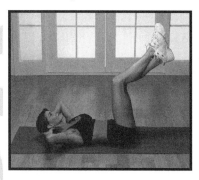 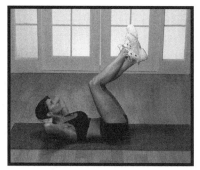

For at home. Lie on a bench or pad. Place your hands at the sides of your head. With your legs up, knees bent slightly, ankles crossed (as shown) keep your eyes on the ceiling and without pulling your head forward perform an abdominal crunch, bringing your knees in at the same time. As you execute this movement, exhale fully and *squeeze* your abdominals. This move works both the upper and lower portions of the abs. It is similar to a crunch combined with a reverse crunch. Do not lower your feet until you complete all the reps. Work within the reps and sets, but if you want to do more, go for it!

SET ONE: 10–15 repetitions
SET TWO: 10–15 repetitions
SET THREE: 10–15 repetitions

HEALTH SMARTS

WHEN DOES FAT BECOME UNHEALTHY?

At what point does being overweight go from unattractive, to irritating, to life threatening? That is not a stupid question but a very serious and complex one. As is the converse: are you so skinny you're risking your life?

Obesity, particularly in our children, has finally been given the high priority it deserves. Obesity is a disease, and there is an epidemic in America. In general, 30 pounds overweight makes you clinically obese. Too many people fall into that category. However, because of body type and bone structure, this general measurement may not be correct.

The problem doesn't end with being too fat. Society's idolization of stick-thin women has messed with our collective mind-set when it comes to our bodies and fat. Even though our intellect tells us that 6% body fat is sickly, many women still believe we can never be too rich or too thin. Thank goodness science has given us some objective measurements to evaluate our body fat and health.

Such assessments have come a long way since I was a kid and we relied on the height-weight chart on the doctor's wall. Of the many means of establishing "healthy" weight today, the best is described below and includes a combination of the Body Mass Index (BMI), the hip-to-waist ratio, and a simple lifestyle checklist.

> **Body mass index:** For those unfamiliar with the term, BMI provides a measure of our body's ratio of fat-to-lean muscle mass. This index is considered superior to others in that it allows for some individuals who may weigh heavy on a height-weight chart but who are carrying more muscle than fat. Although the BMI is an improvement
>
> *continued*

> over most measurements, I feel a more accurate gauge of health requires all three assessments.
>
> The point to remember is that fat isn't just unattractive, it can kill. Being seriously overweight greatly increases the risk of diabetes, hypertension, and other chronic disorders, which can drastically reduce the quality of our lives.

First, calculate your BMI: I have seen several ways to calculate this index, and I find the following formula to be the simplest:

1. Multiply your weight in pounds by 700.
2. Square your height in inches (multiply your height in inches by itself).
3. Divide #1 by #2.

   For example:
   125 pounds x 700 = 87,500
   5'4" = 64 inches x 64 = 4,096
   87,500 ÷ 4,096 = 21.36

A BMI calculated in this manner should be 27 or lower to be in the healthy range. People with a BMI above 27 are considered obese.

Second, check hip-to-waist ratio: While the tendency for women to gain fat disproportionately in the buttocks, hips, and thighs is unattractive, it is actually more healthy than gaining fat in the torso, as most men do. The "apple" shape, which most overweight men possess, has virtually no waist and is more prone to obesity-related diseases than the "pear" shape.

To further determine your health risk, you need to look at your hip-to-waist ratio. Take your girth measurements at your navel and at the widest point of your hips, just over your buttocks. Divide your waist measurement by your hip measurement. For example: a 26-inch waist divided by 38-inch hips equals .68.

For most women, the hip-to-waist ratio should fall below .80 to be considered healthy. For most men, the hip-to-waist ratio should fall below 1.00 to be considered healthy.

Third, review your lifestyle: To further determine health risk, I ask my "patients" the following lifestyle questions:

1. Do you have high blood pressure, diabetes, osteoarthritis, high cholesterol, or high triglycerides?
2. Does anyone in your family have any of these conditions or has anyone had heart disease?

3. Do you smoke cigarettes, overeat, drink more than one alcoholic drink per day, or live with a high degree of stress?

4. Have you gained more than 15 pounds after age 25?

If you answered yes to two or more of the questions above, and if your BMI is more than 27 and your hip-to-waist ratio is high, your health is in serious jeopardy because of your weight. A reduction in weight will begin to lower that risk immediately.

TAKE THIS THOUGHT TO BED WITH YOU

Open up to your logbooks and look at what you've accomplished. Your basic conditioning should be way up on the scale already. Are your thoughts staying positive?

Thousands of people have asked me to help them with their programs. They always start off telling me how they exercise and eat well, but nothing seems to change. As soon as I have them write down everything they ate and did for a week, the problem becomes obvious: they are consuming more calories than they expend. Usually the calories are high-glycemic—the type that stores as fat.

Pretend you're Tony Little and looking at your mom's, daughter's, or husband's logbooks. Using your knowledge, do you see anything wrong? Any missed workouts? Too many substitutions?

Keeping track is the best way to identify and correct errors. If you do the program, it will work.

Good night. Tomorrow's another big and exciting day. You are what you think you are—so be sure to think you're someone really great!

Do it! Write it! Be it!

WHAT YOU ATE (If you swallowed it, write it down)

Breakfast: Lunch: Supper:

_____   _____   _____

_____   _____   _____

_____   _____   _____

_____   _____   _____

_____   _____   _____

_____   _____   _____

_____   _____   _____

_____   _____   _____

Snacks:

WHAT YOU DID

Cardiovascular Exercise	Time	Notes
_____	_____	_____
_____	_____	_____

Resistance Exercise	Reps/Sets/Weight	Notes
_____	_____	_____
_____	_____	_____
_____	_____	_____
_____	_____	_____
_____	_____	_____
_____	_____	_____
_____	_____	_____

WHAT YOU THOUGHT

_____
_____
_____
_____
_____
_____
_____
_____
_____
_____
_____
_____
_____
_____
_____
_____
_____
_____
_____
_____
_____
_____
_____
_____
_____

ONLY 17 DAYS TO GO!

DAY 12

When people think of exercise, they think of work. When I think about exercise, I think about fun and feeling better, sweating out my stress. I also think about rest.

For resistance exercise to work its magic, rest is as important as effort. This means rest between sets (up to one full minute) and a good night's sleep.

A sound night's sleep allows your body to recharge. Certain hormones are released during restful sleep that help regenerate your body and build healthy energetic lean muscle. Spend your day working on getting a good night's rest by taking care of nagging matters, getting all your work done, taking the time to feed and exercise your body well, and bringing a little sunshine and a smile to the lives of those around you. That done, you should sleep like a just-fed puppy.

EATING RIGHT

Food was put on this planet to feed us. Fruits and many vegetables are beautiful plants and flowers that give us enjoyment in the garden. What a great idea to have these eye-pleasers turn into taste-pleasers on our plates and palates.

Try to eat foods that are as close to their natural state as possible. Fresh is nearly always better. They look good on you!

BREAKFAST

Breakfast on the go: Grab a meal replacement prepared drink or bar or soup for breakfast. Drink coffee or tea (no sugar) or hot chocolate and consume a big bottle of water.

Sit-down breakfast: Fix some egg substitute, egg whites, or three egg whites with one egg yolk for you yolk-lovers. Sauté diced bell pepper, diced onion, and finely diced broccoli crowns in a pan coated with Pam, then add the eggs and scramble them alongside the vegetables. Enjoy the scramble with half a cantaloupe and a slice of rye or multi-grain bread with almond-butter spread. Enjoy your coffee, tea, or fat-free milk on the side.

LUNCH

Lunch on the go: I can't recommend most fast foods, but in a real bind, Taco Bell's bean burrito with extra lettuce meets our requirements. Subway's six-inch, under-six-grams-of-fat sandwiches also fill the bill. Be sure to drink lots of water with either one!

Sit-down lunch: Mix up a salad consisting of lettuce, chickpeas, diced cucumber, a medium tomato, and some chopped onion. Add a dressing of a tablespoon of olive oil and a tablespoon of vinegar, with salt and pepper to taste. On the side, have half a sandwich of turkey or chicken deli meat, with lettuce, tomato, and light mayonnaise on rye bread.

Have an apple or orange for dessert. Drink at least eight ounces of water.

SUPPER

Supper on the go: Grab a fist-sized portion of lean meat from the deli and enjoy with a cup of lentil or split pea soup, or a three-bean or pasta salad. Enjoy a low-fat, low-sugar yogurt, preferably plain, with nuts or fresh fruit for dessert.

Sit-down supper: Start with a cup of lentil soup—the low-sodium canned variety. Grill a fist-sized piece of lean fish, beef, or poultry. Bake two one-inch slices of eggplant, glazed with olive oil and topped with mozzarella cheese right out of the oven. Top it off with a scoop of sorbet or fresh fruit medley with Cool Whip for dessert.

Again, drink plenty of water with your meal.

WORKOUT

There will be cardio and more resistance exercise today. Make today count! You get two days of active rest in between. And hey, you can do anything, right?

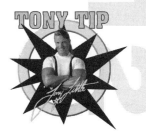

When you eat a certain way, you look a certain way. Want to look like a doughboy? Well, eat the dough, boy! Want to look like a celery stick? Well, you get the hint. You are what you eat!

This holds true when you're eating out. If you walk into a restaurant and see nothing but super-sized people, chances are those super-sized portions are the root of the cause. I'd turn on my heel and head for the place where thin people eat! Or, I'd make certain I had a healthy order in my head before I walked through the door!

CARDIOVASCULAR EXERCISE

From your arsenal of cardio routines, pick one and today invest 25 minutes of your time. Remember to work at a PRE of 6 to 8.

Music always makes the time go faster, so pick a beat that gets your adrenaline pumping! And turn it up *loud!* If you want killer workout music, call me! Or, look on my website! What's more effective than a kick-butt personal trainer and kick-butt music while exercising!

> ## Be sure to keep track of everything
> ## in your logbook!

RESISTANCE EXERCISE

Here we go again! Make the third set count! Today is reserved for maximum calorie burn by hitting the legs heavy, and then some abs to finish things off.

> My recommendations for repetitions are general guidelines. Do more if you can—have a no-limits attitude!

1. Wide-stance squat (legs, inner thighs):

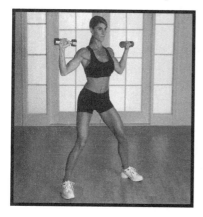 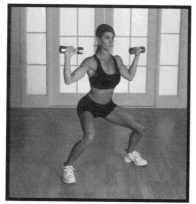

For at home or at the gym. Use your bodyweight or light, 8- to 15-pound dumbbells. Stand with your feet wider apart than shoulder width, toes pointed out at ten and two o'clock. Keep your back straight and your eyes up, and squat down as far as comfortable. Then *squeeze* your glutes!

SET ONE: 10–15 repetitions
SET TWO: 10–15 repetitions
SET THREE: 10–15 repetitions

1a. Leg press machine (quads, hamstrings, inner thighs):

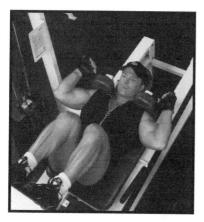 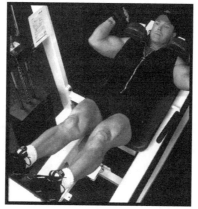

For the gym only. Begin by pushing the platform up past the slide guards. Once you remove these guards, the machine has the capability to come nearly all the way down. Be certain the weight is under your control. With abs, arms, and legs tense, lower the weight as far as comfortable and without allowing the reverse motion and then *squeeze* back to the top. Adjust the weight by checking it first with one rep. It should be comfortable for one set. Concentrate on technique.

SET ONE: 10–15 repetitions
SET TWO: 10–15 repetitions
SET THREE: 10–15 repetitions

2. Stationary lunge (hamstrings, gluteals):

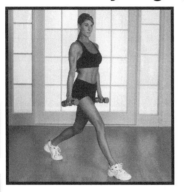 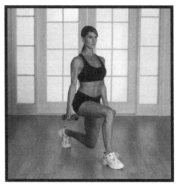

For at home or at the gym. Use only your bodyweight or light, 5- to 15-pound dumbbells. Perform this lunge by standing upright and taking a large stride forward with your right leg. This is the start position. Bending your right knee, let your left knee trail as low as comfortable. Keep your forward knee over the ball of your foot. Stand back up to the start position—think squeeze. Finish all your reps for one leg before moving to the other leg.

SET ONE: 8–10 repetitions per leg
SET TWO: 8–10 repetitions per leg
SET THREE: 8–10 repetitions per leg

2a. Leg extension (quadriceps):

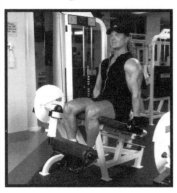 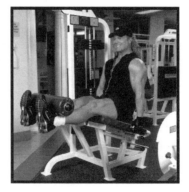

For the gym only. Hold onto the side handles. Squeeze your quads as you extend your legs straight out in front of you. Hold for one second at the peak contraction and squeeze, then lower the bar. Don't go heavy with the weights. Concentrate on technique.

SET ONE: 10–15 repetitions
SET TWO: 10–15 repetitions
SET THREE: 10–15 repetitions

3. Back Row with chair (v-taper of back):

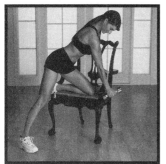 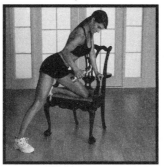 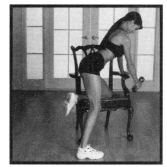

For at home or at the gym. This is a great exercise for strengthening the back. At home, find a sturdy armless chair and kneel on it as shown. In the gym, use a bench. Try and keep your chest almost parallel to the floor and your back straight, balance on the chair with one arm and hold a dumbbell (use a light, 5- to 20-pound dumbbell) at arm's length in the other hand. Keeping your upper body tense, squeeze the dumbbell up to the side of your chest, elbow slightly bent out, then return to arm's length and stretch (but not to the floor).

SET ONE: 10–15 repetitions
SET TWO: 10–15 repetitions

3a. Back row machine (back):

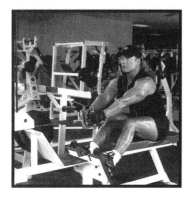 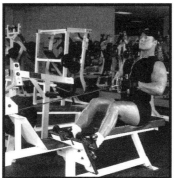

For the gym only. Grab the close-grip handles on a rowing machine with a 45-degree back, then push back with your legs until there is tension on the cable. From this position, pull the handles close to your body and squeeze your shoulder blades at the peak of the movement. Return to the original position. Adjust weight for a good squeeze technique—try to go as heavy as you can. However, make your movements fluid, not jerky.

SET ONE: 10–15 repetitions
SET TWO: 10–15 repetitions

4. Modified push-up or push-up (chest):

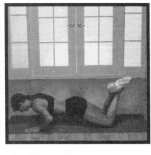
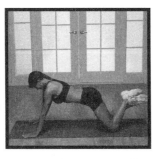
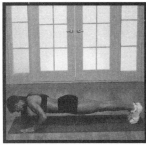
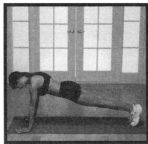

For at home or at the gym. You may perform this according to your conditioning. The easiest way is to perform it leaning against a table-high object. A more difficult push-up may be done lying flat on the floor and pushing up from your knees (as shown). The hardest form of push-up is lying flat on your stomach and pushing your entire body up from the floor while only your hands and toes are touching the floor. In all the different variations, your hands should be positioned just outside your shoulders, arms slightly bent out, elbows in line with your shoulders, back straight and your neck in a neutral position. Lower down to the point just before your chest touches the floor and then squeeze your chest muscles as you raise up, repeat.

SET ONE: 10–15 repetitions
SET TWO: 10–15 repetitions
SET THREE: 10–15 repetitions

4a. Chest press machine (chest):

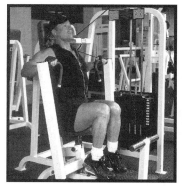 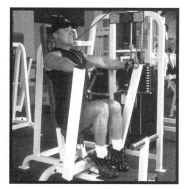

For the gym only. With your feet firmly on the pad, tense your upper body, particularly your chest, and push the weight directly in front of you. Hold for one-half second at the peak contraction, then return to the original position under control. Adjust weight for squeeze technique, not jerky motion.

> **SET ONE:** 10–15 repetitions
> **SET TWO:** 10–15 repetitions
> **SET THREE:** 10–15 repetitions

5. Triceps extension (back of upper arms):

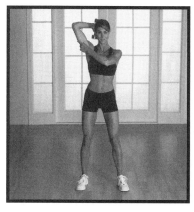 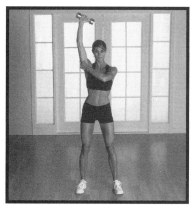

For at home or at the gym. Use a light, 8- to 15-pound dumbbell. You don't want the backs of your arms flapping in the wind. Be sure to keep your upper arm stable and lower the weight as far as comfortable behind your head. Return to the original position.

> **SET ONE:** 10–12 repetitions
> **SET TWO:** 10–12 repetitions

5a. Seated triceps pushdown on machine (back of upper arms):

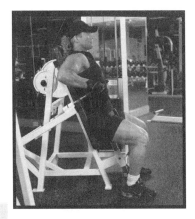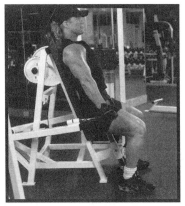

For the gym only. Sit in a triceps pushdown machine and grab both handles. Feet should be solid on the floor. Squeezing your triceps, press the handles down to arms' length. Adjust the weight for fluid squeezing technique. It should not be too heavy.

SET ONE: 10–12 repetitions
SET TWO: 10–12 repetitions

6. Dual bicep curl (biceps):

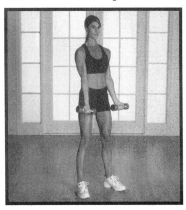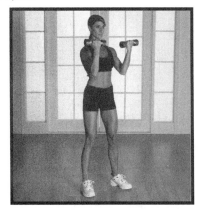

For at home or at the gym. Begin with a dumbbell in each hand, palms forward. *Squeeze* your biceps and abs as you curl the dumbbell up so that your palms are facing your shoulders. Try to start increasing the weight of the dumbbells on this one. For example, if you are using five-pound dumbbells now try moving up to eight-pound ones. The last five reps should be hard to complete. Always use the smallest increments available.

SET ONE: 10–15 repetitions
SET TWO: 10–15 repetitions

6a. Barbell arm curl (biceps):

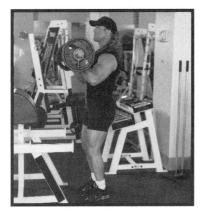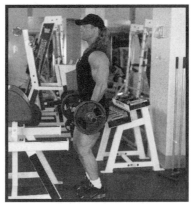

For the gym only. Stand in front of a rack and pick up a barbell in both hands. Make certain your grip is centered, palms facing away from you. Squeeze your biceps hard as you bring the weight up so your palms are facing your chest. Return slowly. Find a weight that is heavy, but still allows you to complete 15 reps with the squeeze at the end!

> **SET ONE:** 10–15 repetitions
> **SET TWO:** 10–15 repetitions

7. Ab crunch (upper abdominals):

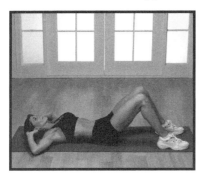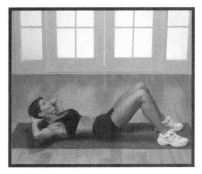

For at home or at the gym. Keep your body as tense as possible and keep these movements slow and precise. Think *squeeze* and technique!

> **SET ONE:** 10–15 repetitions
> **SET TWO:** 10–15 repetitions
> **SET THREE:** 10–12 repetitions

8. Reverse crunch (lower abdominals):

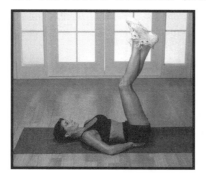 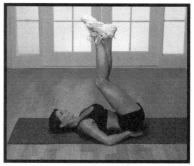

For at home or at the gym. Think squeeze technique! Don't let that lower back come too far off the ground, and breathe out as you bear down on the lower abs.

SET ONE: 10–15 repetitions
SET TWO: 10–15 repetitions
SET THREE: 10–12 repetitions

Finish with some light stretching. See page 301.

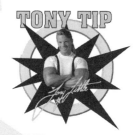

Good things come to those who wait. Don't go jumpin' on that darn scale. Instead, try on the pants or skirt or shorts, and see if they're getting a little less snug or loose as a goose!

HEALTH SMARTS

SLEEP TIGHT, SLEEP RIGHT, LOOK TIGHT!

Insomnia can really mess up your life. If you toss and turn all night, you're not alone. About half of all adults suffer from sleep problems at some point in their lives. Prescription medications do not work in the long run and many are dangerously addictive. Fortunately, there are a number of safe, natural alternatives.

First of all, be sure you make the obvious lifestyle changes before you begin taking supplements for insomnia. These include cutting back (or cutting out completely) caffeine and alcohol. It's ironic that some people use alcohol to help them sleep, because it is far more likely to disturb the quality of sleep, or cause you to wake up in the middle of the night or too early in the morning.

Second, try Mother Nature's remedy for all kinds of ailments—exercise. Exercise is good for insomnia because it makes you feel physically tired, and exhaustion is a great sleep inducer. Just make sure you don't exercise right before bedtime, because exercise initially acts to energize and invigorate you. Give your body several hours after exercise to wind down and prepare for sleep.

Lastly, avoid eating a big, heavy meal before bedtime, because the digestive process can interfere with restful sleep. It may also help to keep your bedroom cool and dark. If after trying these things you are still having trouble falling asleep or waking frequently, try these natural remedies below.

Melatonin for natural sleep inducement: Melatonin is a hormone produced by a tiny, pea-sized gland in the brain called the pineal gland. This hormone controls circadian rhythm—our internal body clock that tells us when to go to sleep and when to wake up. Besides regulating our sleep cycles, melatonin is thought to have potent anti-aging properties.

The problem is that our melatonin levels peak during childhood; then, when other hormones start to kick in during our teen years, melatonin levels drop and continue to decrease as we age. In fact, by the time we reach age 60, our melatonin level is about half of what it was at age 20.

Research reveals that taking melatonin supplements in low doses (approximately 1 to 3 mg. before bedtime) is safe for adults and will help restore restful sleep patterns within a few days to a few weeks. Always check with your physician before taking any herbal supplement.

Sleepytime supplements vitamin B$_{12}$ and calcium: Vitamin B$_{12}$ may help overcome insomnia because it aids in the production of melatonin. Since there is also an age-related decline in this essential vitamin, taking supplements can be beneficial. They are best taken as part of a multivitamin supplement. Many multivitamin supplements are available now by sex and age to give you a safe but effective dose.

Although it's usually not a good idea to take vitamin/mineral supplements before bed, calcium is the exception—it's a potent sleep inducer. Try taking supplements at least a half-hour before bedtime for a calming effect on the body.

Herbal teas: Chamomile tea has been a popular antidote for sleeplessness for centuries. Two other herbs, valerian and kava kava, are also very effective when used as a tea. Valerian root can also help ease stress and act as a mental relaxant. Both valerian and kava kava are also available in capsule form.

I recommend over-the-counter or prescription sleeping aids and tranquilizers only as a last resort, and only for short periods of time. Although these drugs may initially knock you out, you'll probably wake up groggy with a "hangover" the next day. I encourage you to try natural remedies. They really work!

TAKE THIS THOUGHT TO BED WITH YOU

Take a little physical inventory tonight. You've had an incredibly big week of workouts—à la champion status, I'd say.

Get in front of the mirror tonight. Be a ham, flex your muscles (four of the thighs). Look at your body and know your doing the best thing you've ever done for yourself!

Doesn't your body feel good? And don't you feel good to be in your body?

Pleasant dreams to a person who deserves nothing less.

DAY 12

Do it! Write it! Be it!

WHAT YOU ATE (If you swallowed it, write it down)

Breakfast: Lunch: Supper:

_____   _____   _____

_____   _____   _____

_____   _____   _____

_____   _____   _____

_____   _____   _____

_____   _____   _____

_____   _____   _____

Snacks:

WHAT YOU DID

Cardiovascular Exercise   Time   Notes

_____   _____   _____

_____   _____   _____

Resistance Exercise   Reps/Sets/Weight   Notes

_____   _____   _____

_____   _____   _____

_____   _____   _____

_____   _____   _____

_____   _____   _____

_____   _____   _____

_____   _____   _____

WHAT YOU THOUGHT

ONLY 16 DAYS TO GO!

DAY 13

BRAIN POWER

For most of you, the weekend's here. I love the ocean, I love the mountains, fresh air, blue skies, and being outside. That's what weekends are for; so, whether it's sunshiny or gloomy, dress the part and get out and enjoy this beautiful world we live in.

Have you ever thought how simple it would be to stay more active if every day you had a reason to get up and go outside? Take a walk, find walking friends, or help an elderly person get their pet out for a morning walk. Find a tea-time neighbor (several blocks away), walk back and forth to lunch from work, take sunset strolls, and while you're at it, stop and smell the roses.

If we all got back to the simple things of life—instead of getting caught up in all the laziness of modern-day gadgets like phones, TVs, videos, and computers—we probably wouldn't be having this epidemic of obesity.

EATING RIGHT

When life hands you lemons, make lemonade! If you're having trouble drinking all the water, water, water I keep talking about, then it's time to get more creative. Lemonade is a starter. So is iced tea, but not the Southern sweet tea. Mineral water (low in sodium) with a dash of 100% fruit juice is always a winner. The bubbles always make it feel like a special drink!

The grocery stores and health food aisles are filled with alternatives to plain water. Explore. Crystal Light or fruit-flavored waters are wonderful. Be sure that the calories aren't over 150 a serving and the sodium is not over 300 mg.!

BREAKFAST

Breakfast on the go: The best quick breakfast in the world is a homemade smoothie made with extra low-carbohydrate protein, Yoplait light yogurt, fresh fruit, nonfat milk, and lots of ice. Grab, gulp, and go!

Sit-down breakfast: Try a healthy, high-carbohydrate meal for slow-burning energy all day long of a half-cup of slow-cooked oats (or low-fat, low-sodium, high-fiber cereal) with berries, nuts, and nonfat milk. Also have a scoop of protein powder mixed with low-fat, low-sugar yogurt, preferably plain, coffee or tea, and all the water you want.

You're loaded with high-energy carbohydrates, so get out and enjoy the day!

LUNCH

Lunch on the go: Head to a salad bar (not a buffet line) for lots of greens and vegetables, tuna, chicken, or egg for protein; and two tablespoons of your favorite dressing. Have some rye crackers with your salad and a diet soda or all the water you can drink.

Sit-down lunch: Either make its equivalent at home, or go out for a chunky chicken salad, fajita salad (without the sour cream), chef's salad, or Cobb salad (without the bacon and blue cheese). Keep dressings on the side and limit them to no more than two tablespoons. Enjoy a cup of lentil, barley, or vegetable soup. And drink lots of water!

SUPPER

Supper on the go: Have a meal replacement bar or shake with nutty trail mix, low-fat yogurt, preferably plain, a piece of fruit, and plenty of water.

Sit-down supper: Choose a lean protein source, then check the list of low-glycemic carbohydrates for a vegetable and a carbohydrate. Fix proper proportions for yourself and enjoy. Or, take yourself out to a restaurant and request selections from your list.

Always drink plenty of water with your meals. Water helps you reach that full feeling sooner. Sorbet or fresh fruit for dessert are great.

WORKOUT

Remember active rest? That's getting outdoors and moving. Put a star on your calendar for every day you get out and do a little bit more than usual.

So, if you walk your dog every day, that doesn't count for a gold star. If you walk your dog twice as far, it does. Go the extra distance and mark your calendar. Soon enough, you'll see so many stars you won't want the stars to stop!

Putting stars on your calendar for every good workout day sounds silly, and maybe even a little stupid. But real stupidity is having a national obesity epidemic, when all the tools to good health and nutrition are at our fingertips!

Come on. Be a little silly. It keeps us young.

CARDIOVASCULAR EXERCISE

Put in 30 minutes of cardio today. Either choose one of your favorites from the previous days, or be creative. Take a hike. Ride a bike. Keep up one activity for 30 minutes today, and do it with a smile! While there are no resistance moves today, you should put in 15 minutes of stretching.

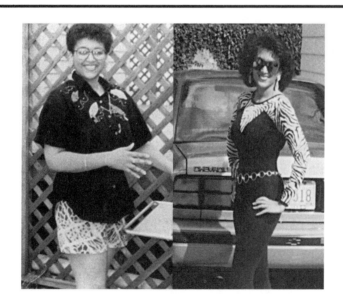

Marla Pluck from Ohio kept her logs and stuck to her program, lost 27 pounds and looks terrific!

MEAL REPLACEMENTS: AN EASY KEY TO WEIGHT LOSS

Several years back the FDA cracked down on manufacturers for calling nutritional drinks and bars "meal replacements." Certainly the term implies that you can replace meals with these protein-enriched drinks and nutrient bars, and that isn't entirely so. When used properly, and not as your sole nutrient source, however, these can indeed replace a meal here and there and get you started on a weight loss program, or supplement the nutrition needed for your athletic pursuits.

Because there are people who think they can survive on meal replacements alone we must use the term carefully—thus my repeated warnings to *use meal replacements no more than twice a day.*

A perfect source of protein: Protein, in a natural diet, is tough to get without increasing the bad dietary saturated fats as well. Therefore, protein-enriched drinks and nutrient bars are great for both dieters and athletes. In general, men have higher protein requirements than women. So do most athletes, especially those involved in bodybuilding. Check that the drink or bar you choose is rich in high-quality protein. This is often referred to as "complete" protein, meaning the food has all the amino acids needed for assimilation. If you are lactose intolerant, seek out a whey protein or soy protein.

The sugar vs. taste dilemma: Next, check that the sugar content, particularly simple sugars, is relatively low. Drinking your vitamins, minerals, and protein in a fructose-flavored syrup or a sugar-laden dough is not going to do your body good.

The reason some nutritional drinks are loaded with sugar is to improve the taste. Yes, sugar tastes good. If you are using one of these drinks for therapeutic reasons—to supplement your energy stores or enable you to lose weight—then I suggest you try out the not-so-tasty low-sugar varieties. If you are simply looking for a nutritionally balanced food source to replace that fast-food burger or hastily prepared tide-me-over snack, then indulge in some sugar. You're still better off than the high-fat alternative.

The additives: What distinguishes high-protein drinks and nutritional bars from sugarcoated wastes of money is their content of superior and highly specific supplements. Creatine- and/or glutamine-enriched powders have proven to be an athlete's best friend.

If you're a woman, seek out low-sugar drinks providing no more than 20% of your protein RDA per serving. Look for formulas that contain little or no maltodextrin, or glycerin, both hidden forms of bad carbohydrates (high-glycemic carbohydrates destined for fat storage). Ingredients are listed in order of the quantity a food contains, so last is least. Also look for weight loss enhancers such as pyruvate, carnitine, lysine, arginine, and chromium picolinate.

Everyone should seek out calcium-containing supplements and those with both soluble and insoluble fiber. As a general rule, powder drink mixes are better than premixed drinks because they contain fewer preservatives and chemicals, and higher-quality nutrients.

How to use: High-protein drinks and nutritional bars are great when you are in a hurry or otherwise unable to prepare a healthy, fresh meal. That's why I use them as my on-the-go meals. Definitely reach for a drink or a nutritional bar instead of fast food. Same goes for sugar cravings—even the high-sugar drinks and bars are nutritionally better for you than candy.

If you're trying to cut calories, these supplements are a great way to ensure optimum nutrition, even though you're decreasing caloric consumption. If you suffer from chocolate cravings, find a healthful drink or bar that satisfies that same craving—chocolate is the most popular flavor in these supplements!

TAKE THIS THOUGHT TO BED WITH YOU

The greatest tragedy is not death but what dies in you while you're still living.

Did you find a fun activity to do today? Next time you're looking for fun, how about rediscovering something that you've dropped from your daily agenda? Too often sedentary living comes about not from necessity but from simply forgetting to keep doing the things we enjoy.

When you fall asleep tonight, think back to the physical things that used to give you so much pleasure. Dream about them. Tomorrow, perhaps you'll do them.

Sleep well.

Do it! Write it! Be it!

WHAT YOU ATE (If you swallowed it, write it down)

Breakfast: Lunch: Supper:

_____ _____ _____
_____ _____ _____
_____ _____ _____
_____ _____ _____
_____ _____ _____
_____ _____ _____
_____ _____ _____

Snacks:

WHAT YOU DID

Cardiovascular Exercise   Time   Notes

_____ _____ _____
_____ _____ _____
_____ _____ _____
_____ _____ _____

Other Activities

_____
_____
_____
_____
_____
_____
_____
_____

WHAT YOU THOUGHT

_____
_____
_____
_____
_____
_____
_____
_____
_____
_____
_____
_____
_____
_____
_____
_____
_____
_____
_____
_____
_____
_____
_____
_____
_____

ONLY 15 DAYS TO GO!

DAY 14

BRAIN POWER

As they say, when one door closes, another door opens.

Today we close the door on week two. What an accomplishment! That means tomorrow you are more than halfway through! And feeling good and looking good!

Way to go, trainee!

Spend today reflecting back on the last two weeks. Review your logbooks and reinforce the progress you've made. Remember when ten minutes of cardio seemed like an eternity? Well, now you're practically the energy bunny.

Be patient. The habit is growing. And remember that even though the grass looks greener on the other side of the fence, it still has to be mowed!

You'll get there. Just stick with me. One step at a time.

EATING RIGHT

Never, ever use starvation diets. Small, frequent meals are the answer. Feed yourself when you're hungry—but be sure to feed yourself with energy foods that are high in protein or low on the Glycemic Index. But for heaven's sake, do feed yourself!

Obey your thirst. Always drink when you're thirsty. Get in the habit of carrying bottled water with you everywhere. Obey your hunger. Eat when you're hungry. Denying yourself food just makes your body hold on to its fat stores harder than ever!

BREAKFAST

Breakfast on the go: You know what to reach for. Meal replacements with a serving of lowfat yogurt, preferably plain, a piece of fruit, or a light salad as a complement. Plus, plenty of water!

Sit-down breakfast: Increase your protein for some good brain food and start out with a nice slice of lean ground turkey, egg substitutes, or a soy burger. Add a side of cottage cheese and two pieces of rye toast with an all-fruit spread or almond butter. Finish it off with sliced apple or apricots. Be sure to drink at least one glass of water, nonfat milk or tea or coffee with your meal.

LUNCH

Lunch on the go: Prepare yourself a Lean Cuisine, Healthy Choice, or Weight Watchers high-protein frozen meal with a piece of fruit and plenty of water!

Sit-down lunch: Have two slices of sourdough, whole-grain, or rye bread with some lean meat or grilled portobello mushroom, a dab of mayonnaise, a slice of avocado, some lettuce or sprouts, and a slice of tomato.

SUPPER

Supper on the go: Go for a meal replacement drink and a baked potato with cheese and salsa or A-1 sauce. Have some fruit and—you guessed it!—lots of water!

Sit-down supper: Indulge yourself a little. Choose a generous fist-sized portion of lean meat or another source of protein, and have this with a fist-sized portion of vegetables and low-glycemic carbohydrate. Finish the meal with low-fat, low-sugar yogurt, preferably plain mixed with nuts and your favorite fruit. Don't forget to drink plenty of water.

If it's still two hours before bedtime, go to your newly stocked cupboards and find yourself a late night snack that pleases your palate.

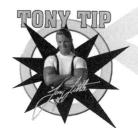

WORKOUT

As with yesterday, today is an active rest day. Chores are always a Sunday favorite—whether in the yard or in the house. Be sure to take some time for rest today as well.

De-stress with a massage, a long bath, a good book, or an hour on the porch swing thinking about the progress you've made. Or do some stretches, and meditation in the morning.

Don't forget that rest is as important as action in a balanced program of healthy fitness for life.

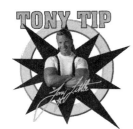

Find a new type of water to enjoy: spend at least a half-hour in the water, in the form of a long shower, bath, hot tub, or swim.

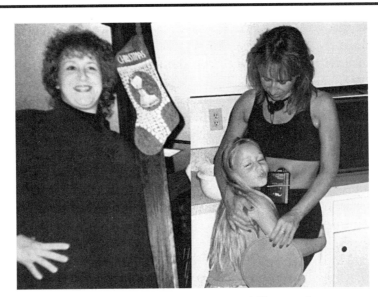

Use the tape measure, not the scale.
Diann Rapps from Missouri lost 62 inches
on her program (that's more than five feet!).
What a good role model!

HEALTH SMARTS

WATER: A MIRACLE FOR WEIGHT LOSS

On average, a human being can survive only three hours in extreme weather with no shelter, three days with no water, and three weeks with no food. I've heard this called the 3-3-3 rule and I remind my friends of it when they go camping in the desert. I also use it to remind people how incredibly important it is to hydrate themselves constantly, throughout the day, every day of their lives.

Water is your best source of hydration. Even if you don't buy into the eight-glasses-a-day theory (which, by the way, has never been proven), you can obtain water from nearly every food source, with fruits and vegetables providing the most. Next are the many types of drinks you may enjoy, but some of these are better than others:

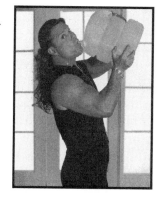

- ▶ Distilled water: Great for short-term use and lessening water retention.
- ▶ Bottled water and spring water: Can contain high levels of sodium; check consumer sources to be sure of quality.
- ▶ Milk: Except for nonfat and 1%, contains high saturated fat and calorie content.
- ▶ Sport drinks: One of the nicest alternatives; read labels carefully for low calories, low sodium, low sugar, and nutritious additives.
- ▶ Tap water: Fine, as long as it comes from a municipal system and is not contaminated; may be fluoridated for stronger bones and teeth.
- ▶ Fruit juices: Healthy, yes, but loaded with simple sugars and calories.
- ▶ Crystal Light: A dieter's delight—zero calories and plenty of flavor.
- ▶ Iced tea: Healthy, if you don't add sugar; try making it with raspberry tea. Green tea makes a great iced tea with added health benefits.
- ▶ Flavored waters: Check calories and sodium content, but usually these clear fruit-flavored drinks are healthy and very low in calories.
- ▶ Diet sodas: Contain additives and sugar substitutes that may carry some health risks; many contain caffeine, but are better than regular sodas!
- ▶ Coffee: Okay in the morning but caffeine has a dehydrating effect so if you drink coffee be sure to drink lots of water too!
- ▶ Alcoholic drinks: An occasional glass of wine or other beverage is okay, but limit your intake.

Hydration and Weight Loss

The fact that you can die in three days with no fluid should be reason enough to drink lots of fluids. However, there are quite a few other good reasons. Hydration helps revitalize cells, flushes some pollutants from your body, contributes to clearer complexions, and improves digestion and bowel movements.

For the person trying to lose weight, water acts as a catalyst to utilize nutrients optimally so that even when calories are reduced, health is maintained.

Water also gives a feeling of fullness. This has been proven in scientific studies to prevent people from reaching for seconds as well as to eat less throughout the day. It's the first and simplest step you should take on your way to accomplishing your weight loss goals.

Remember, it's easy to sweat away more than a quart of water during an hour of exercise, especially in hot weather. During extremely strenuous exercise, athletes have sweat rates of nearly a gallon an hour.

Obviously, when you exercise you must hydrate yourself. Water is best, though special sport drinks, or diluted fruit juice, which contain a little sugar and sodium, may be okay during some strenuous exercise.

Hydrate yourself before, during, and after exercise. Drink even if you don't feel thirsty. Realize, if you live an active life in a warm climate, it's recommended that you drink at least 16 to 20 ounces of fluid two hours before exercising, another eight ounces 15 to 30 minutes after exercising, and 4 to 6 ounces during every 15 to 20 minutes of exercise.

Have an event you want to look good for? Try my distilled water trick. For two to three weeks prior to the event, drink as much distilled water as possible. Because there are no minerals this tends to help you drop water weight. Be sure to use a good vitamin/mineral supplement when you're limiting your fluids to distilled water.

TAKE THIS THOUGHT TO BED WITH YOU

Your environment continually influences you. Try to put yourself among people who have your best interests in mind. Try to eliminate negatives from your life.

You have embarked on this program. You are proceeding and succeeding. If there is a roadblock ahead, take a different road.

Stay positive and surround yourself with others who are positive as well. You're going to make it.

Stay strong.

Do it! Write it! Be it!

WHAT YOU ATE (If you swallowed it, write it down)

Breakfast: Lunch: Supper:

_____   _____   _____
_____   _____   _____
_____   _____   _____
_____   _____   _____
_____   _____   _____
_____   _____   _____
_____   _____   _____
_____   _____   _____

Snacks:

WHAT YOU DID

Cardiovascular Exercise   Time   Notes

_____   _____   _____
_____   _____   _____
_____   _____   _____
_____   _____   _____

Other Activities

_____
_____
_____
_____
_____
_____
_____
_____

WHAT YOU THOUGHT

_____
_____
_____
_____
_____
_____
_____
_____
_____
_____
_____
_____
_____
_____
_____
_____
_____
_____
_____
_____
_____
_____
_____
_____
_____
_____
_____
_____
_____

ONLY 14 DAYS TO GO!

WEEK 3:
On Track

4

> Terrific job!
>
> It's hard to believe that two short weeks ago you were just embarking on this exciting journey. You've got to admit, it feels great *after* the exercise, doesn't it? That's because your body was made to move and your muscles were made to flex.

DAY 15

BRAIN POWER

They're thanking you for giving them what they need, for pushing fresh new blood deep within the tissues, and for feeding your body with vital nutrients.

If you treat your body well, it won't let you down. Your body is like your vehicle. Do regular maintenance and it won't break down. It will run faster and perform better and won't stall or sputter.

Have you got *it* yet? If not, you should soon. *It* is the positive mentality shared by all people who take care of themselves by exercising and making healthy food choices. It gives us power to make the right decisions about our destiny. It makes us stand taller and walk with more pride.

It begins when you feel just a little more comfortable in your own skin. By taking control of your health and your shape, you are mentally reprogramming yourself to be a positive, decisive individual.

Think positive. You can do anything if you believe you can!

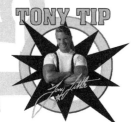

TONY TIP

Your body will adapt to anything—good or bad. Adapt it to the good things.

> ## When life throws you a curve ball, avoid it and let it go. Every minute of every day you have another chance.

EATING RIGHT

Everything you're learning is great for conversation starters at a party. But when it comes to good nutrition, it all boils down to only four things, but they are four *big* things:

1. Eat more frequently
2. Eat smaller portions
3. Increase your activity
4. Drink plenty of water

> **F**ad diets don't work in the long term. They nearly always result in more weight gain when stopped (the yo-yo syndrome.) That's why we see the same old diet gurus producing new books and sequels every decade.

BREAKFAST

Breakfast on the go: A good vitamin/mineral supplement should start your day, every day. If you're rushing out the door, grab that high-protein, low-carbohydrate meal replacement smoothie or bar. The beauty of some of these bars is the fact that they are so dry you'll want to drink at least eight ounces of water with it.

Sit-down breakfast: Have a fist-sized portion of turkey bacon or sliced deli meat, plus low-fat yogurt, preferably plain, or cottage cheese served with walnuts and blueberries, rye bread, and a big glass of skim milk. You can also have coffee or tea, no sugar, black or with a low-fat cream substitute.

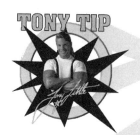

Think ahead and cut up some bite-sized wedges of oranges, melons, celery, or carrot sticks. Or keep some grapes or berries on hand. Having these on hand at home and at work to munch on throughout the day will keep your hunger satisfied.

LUNCH

Lunch on the go: Reach for a meal replacement bar or get a chicken or beef burrito, without the burrito! Just ask them to put the insides in a to-go cup, and hold the sour cream. Pick up a big bottle of spring water.

Sit-down lunch: Add a small amount of low-fat mayonnaise to a can of tuna or chicken, mix with peas and/or chopped celery, and spread on two slices of rye or pumpernickel bread. Add lettuce or sprouts and a little spicy mustard or pickle relish to taste.

Have dried, canned, or fresh apricots for dessert. Drink at least eight ounces of water.

SUPPER

Supper on the go: Hold the mayonnaise on a deli sandwich of either chicken or turkey. Wash it down with a berry smoothie or, of course, water.

Sit-down supper: Have a fist-sized portion of chicken, fish, lean beef, or soy with a fist-sized portion of beans, pasta, noodles, or rice. Add a fist-sized portion of green peas, corn, green beans, raw carrots, or spinach. Enjoy trail mix with nuts and dried fruit for dessert. But don't get the type with carob and yogurt chips—just plain nuts and fruits. And have lots of water!

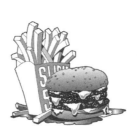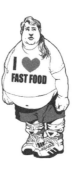

Biggie fries and super sizes will super size you!
Illustration by Matt Gouig

Just remember this: If some fast-food chain promises you a super size, that's exactly what you'll become: a super size! And remember, biggie rhymes with piggy. Instead of supersized colas, how about supersized water!

WORKOUT

We're going to really work you this week. Some of the exercises you know, plus there are some new moves. We've also mixed things up a bit. Here's the drill for the rest of the program: six days cardio, three days resistance, plus two extra ab days. Let's get started.

Before doing any particular exercise, mentally rehearse it in your mind. You can actually do the movements with no weights, just by tensing (squeezing) your muscles as you go through the motions. Mind and muscle have a relationship—strengthen the bond with the squeeze method!

CARDIOVASCULAR EXERCISE

We're in our third week and that means 30 minutes, or more, of continuous, nonstop cardio activity. If age or conditioning makes 30 minutes seem like a life sentence, cut this down to two 15-minute sessions or two 20-minute sessions.

Choose one of your favorite cardio activities. Now, let's rev it up. Begin by marching in place at an easy pace for five minutes. Then do some light stretches. Watch the clock, and now speed your pace up a notch at 15-second intervals, until you are breathing hard. Remember: keep movements fluid, energized, and brisk—not fast, just comfortable. If you feel you're breathing too hard, check your Target Heart Rate (see page 96). After this, proceed with your favorite cardio activity for the duration of the half-hour. Oh yeah, don't count your five-minute warm-up in the total!

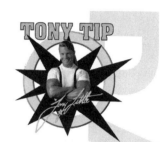

It might be time to expand on your aerobic activities. How about an aerobic tape? There are literally hundreds to choose from. Or, consider joining an aerobic class at a local gym, community college, or community center like the YMCA.

Although each individual is different, on average a person reaches their optimum fat-burning zone within 20 minutes of beginning cardio exercise. At approximately 45 minutes the fat-burning factor of cardio exercises begins to diminish but heart conditioning continues. Bottom line: for weight loss you're better off with 30 to 45 minutes of cardio than with 60! Age and conditioning may make shorter periods better for you.

RESISTANCE EXERCISE

Here we go again. A different arrangement of the exercises you've already learned, plus some new ones to tone you up and lean you out! Resistance exercise is about increasing the workload. More reps equals more resistance. Have you upped the reps or resistance? Go back now and check your logbooks to see how far you've come. You will become ultimately what you do.

For this workout at home you will need some light, 3-, 5-, 8-, 10- and 12-pound dumbbells.

Tempo, the rate of speed at which you perform an exercise, is a critical component of how the exercise affects your muscles. Ideally, strive for a slow concentric movement (the lifting portion) and a slightly faster eccentric movement (the return).

1. Reverse crunches (midsection):

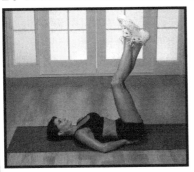 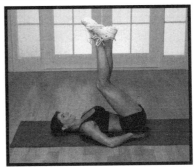

For at home or at the gym. Think squeeze technique! Don't let that lower back come too far off the ground, and breathe out as you bear down on the lower abs.

SET ONE: 10–15 repetitions
SET TWO: 10–15 repetitions
SET THREE: 10–15 repetitions

2. Oblique crunch (front and side midsection):

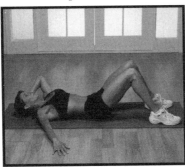 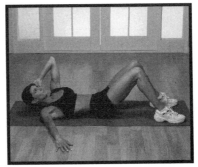

For at home or at the gym. This move works both the abs and the obliques—the large muscles that run down the sides of your torso. Lie on a mat. Place one hand at the side of your head. Knees should be bent and feet flat on the floor. Without pulling your head forward, perform an abdominal crunch with your chin up, pulling your left elbow and shoulder toward your right knee. Alternate with your right elbow and shoulder pulling toward your left knee. Remember to squeeze and hold and do all reps on one side before doing the opposite side.

SET ONE: 10–15 repetitions
SET TWO: 10–15 repetitions
SET THREE: 10–15 repetitions

3. Ab crunches (midsection):

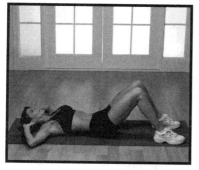 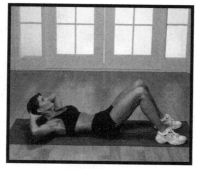

For at home or at the gym. Keep your body as tense as possible and keep these movements slow and precise. Think *squeeze* and technique! For great variety, perform these on a large exercise ball.

SET ONE: 10–15 repetitions
SET TWO: 10–15 repetitions
SET THREE: 10–15 repetitions

4. Full squat (quads, hamstrings, gluteals):

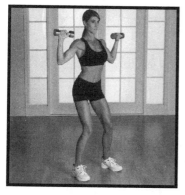 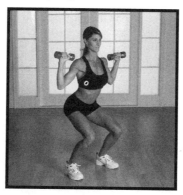

For at home or at the gym. Use your bodyweight or medium (10- to 20-pound) dumbbells. Place your feet shoulder-width apart. If you are using dumbbells, grab two and hold, palms facing forward at your shoulders. The dumbbells remain in this position. Now squat down, keeping your back straight, your chin up, and your rear end sticking out as though you were about to sit in a chair. Try to come all the way down until your upper legs are parallel to the floor. Never go all the way down. You may need to place a book under your heels to elevate them and remove the strain on the Achilles tendon.

SET ONE: 10–15 repetitions
SET TWO: 10–15 repetitions
SET THREE: 10–15 repetitions

DAY 15

4a. Leg press machine (quads, gluteals):

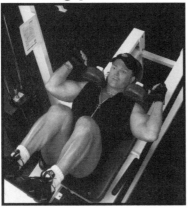 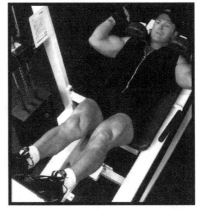

For the gym only. Position the machine so that your knees are bent and you're a little squished at the start. The first portion of this exercise hits the glutes and produces a great-looking butt! Push your legs out until they are straight, but don't lock the knees. Then return, under control, to the start. Machines vary, so experiment with the poundage—you might be a lot stronger on this than you think! Concentrate on squeezing, with no jerky movements. You should be able to do much heavier weight in this machine than on a freestanding squat. Go for it!

SET ONE: 10–15 repetitions
SET TWO: 10–15 repetitions
SET THREE: 10–15 repetitions

5. Back Row with chair (v-taper of back):

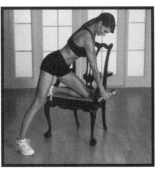 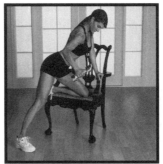 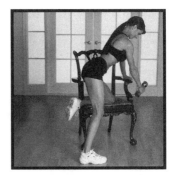

For at home or at the gym. This is a great exercise for strengthening the back. At home, find a sturdy armless chair and kneel on it as shown. In the gym, use a bench. Try and keep your chest almost parallel to the floor and your back straight, balance on the chair with one arm and hold a dumbbell (use a light, 5- to 20-pound dumbbell) at arm's length in the other hand. Keeping your upper body tense, squeeze the dumbbell up to the side of your chest, elbow slightly bent out, then return to arm's length and stretch (but not to the floor).

SET ONE: 10–15 repetitions
SET TWO: 10–15 repetitions
SET THREE: 10–15 repetitions

5a. Back row machine (back):

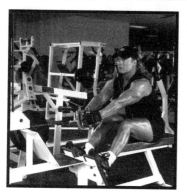 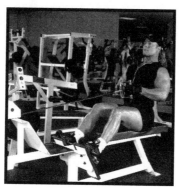

For the gym only. Grab the close-grip handles on a rowing machine with a 45-degree back, then push back with your legs until there is tension on the cable. From this position, pull the handles close to your body and squeeze your shoulder blades at the peak of the movement. Return to the original position and stretch. Concentrate on the squeeze technique, not using heavy weights. Find a weight that is confortable to perform 15 reps with good exercise form and squeezing technique.

SET ONE: 10–15 repetitions
SET TWO: 10–15 repetitions
SET THREE: 10–15 repetitions

6. Chest crossovers (chest):

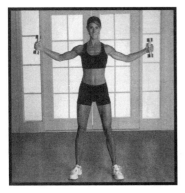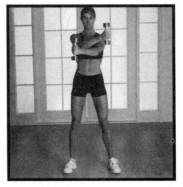

For at home or at the gym. Hold a light, 5- to 15-pound dumbbell in each hand, arms outstretched to your sides. Tighten your abs (core muscles) and bend knees slightly. As though you were hugging a barrel, bring the dumbbells together simultaneously in front of you, then cross and squeeze. You can alternate which arm is on top. *Squeeze*, and return to the original position.

SET ONE: 10–15 repetitions
SET TWO: 10–15 repetitions
SET THREE: 10–15 repetitions

6a. Chest machine or pec deck (chest):

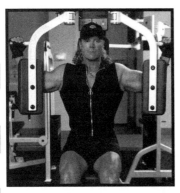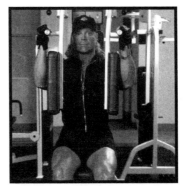

For the gym only. Position the seat so that your forearms are firmly against the pads. With a light grip on the handles squeeze down on your chest muscles and bring the handles together in front of you. Hold for a moment (squeezing) and return to the start for another repetition. Do not let the weights drop—return to start with a bang. This exercise works the inside of the chest, or the cleavage. Caution: never extend your elbows behind your shoulders. Technique is really important, not using a heavy weight.

SET ONE: 10–15 repetitions
SET TWO: 10–15 repetitions
SET THREE: 10–15 repetitions

7. Side lateral (shoulders):

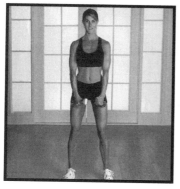 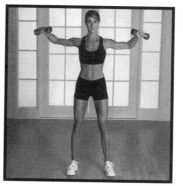

Stand with your feet shoulder-width apart and hold a light, 5- to 12-pound dumbbell in each hand, arms extended to the floor. Tighten abs (core muscles). In an arc, bring the dumbbells up and *squeeze*. Keep your elbows slightly bent throughout the movement and your palms facing down. Return weights to start position with control. You need to raise the dumbbells only slightly above shoulder height.

SET ONE: 10–12 repetitions
SET TWO: 10–12 repetitions
SET THREE: 10–12 repetitions

7a. Lateral cable raise (shoulders):

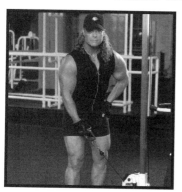 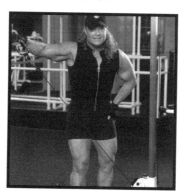

For the gym only. Begin standing alongside a low cable with a single handle. Pick up the handle and stand erect. Tighten abs. In a fluid motion, raise the cable out away from your body to shoulder height. Pause, then return slowly. Remember to *squeeze.* Adjust weight to very light. This really works the side of your deltoids. When done with one side, reverse position and repeat for the other.

SET ONE: 10–12 repetitions
SET TWO: 10–12 repetitions
SET THREE: 10–12 repetitions

8. Triceps kickback (triceps):

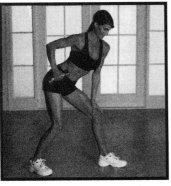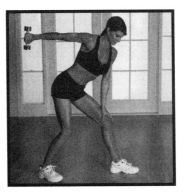

For at home or at the gym. This exercise is great for toning up the backs of the arms. Like the back row, begin by bending as shown and using one hand on your knee for support. With a light, 5- to 15-pound dumbbell at arm's length at your side, bend at the elbow and bring your upper arm up (as shown). This is the start position. Do not move that upper arm! To perform, simply "kick back" your hand and forearm so your arm is straight. Really put the squeeze on the triceps through-out the movement! After all sets are completed, reverse position and repeat for the other side.

SET ONE: 10–12 repetitions
SET TWO: 10–12 repetitions
SET THREE: 10–12 repetitions

DAY 15

8a. Seated triceps extension (triceps):

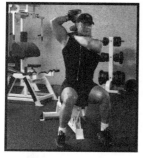 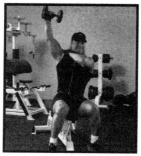

For the gym only. Sit at the end of a bench and hold a dumbbell (as shown) behind your head. Use your other arm to help stabilize the lifting arm and keep the upper arm in the same position as you raise the dumbbell to arm's length. Keep your inner elbow facing forward and *squeeze* at the peak of motion. Return to the original position. Repeat until all reps are done on one side, then switch to the other side.

SET ONE: 10–12 repetitions
SET TWO: 10–12 repetitions
SET THREE: 10–12 repetitions

9. Alternating biceps curl (biceps):

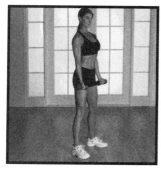 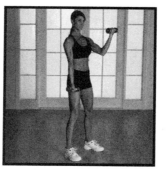

For at home or at the gym. Begin with a medium, 10- to 20-pound dumbbell in each hand, palms forward. *Squeeze* your biceps and abs as you curl the dumbbell up so that your palms are facing your shoulders. Begin with the right arm, then alternate with the left. Get a good rhythm going by starting with the left just as you are about to finish with the right. But never, ever "rock" or swing your body to accomplish the lift. That's cheating! Cheating not only reduces the effect of the exercise, but also can cause injury.

SET ONE: 10–12 repetitions
SET TWO: 10–12 repetitions
SET THREE: 10–12 repetitions

DAY 15

9a. Seated dumbbell curl (biceps):

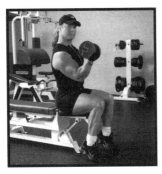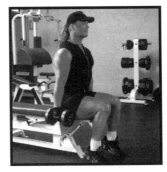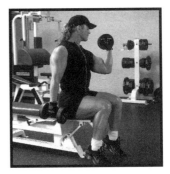

For the gym only. Begin with a heavy, 12- to 30-pound dumbbell in each hand, palms facing you. *Squeeze* your biceps and abs as you curl the dumbbell up so that your palms are facing your shoulders. Begin with the right arm, then alternate with the left. Give the biceps a good squeeze at the top of the movement. Return slowly to start position. Technique is more important than weight.

SET ONE: 10–12 repetitions
SET TWO: 10–12 repetitions
SET THREE: 10–12 repetitions

Finish off with light stretching.

HEALTH SMARTS

FIBER: THE FORGOTTEN NUTRIENT

It took only about 150 years for American ingenuity to destroy the nutritional wealth of this nation. The mass production of foods has removed nearly all the natural nutrients, and in the process, only a scant few have been replaced.

One absolutely necessary nutrient that has virtually disappeared is the fiber found abundantly in whole grains. You may think, "Whoa! I eat my Wheaties, Grape Nuts, or granola." But if you read the label you will find wheat flours and oat flours make up the primary ingredients. The only grains that rate high on a fiber scale are whole grains, and that is what you need to look for on labels. Whole wheat and oatmeal are whole grains; however, oatmeal bread and whole-wheat crackers are not.

Most people know that a high-fiber diet is good for the colon. It helps to keep bowel movements regular because of the insoluble nature of some fiber. But there is also a soluble side of fiber that may have equally important health benefits. Studies have indicated that soluble fiber can attach itself to cholesterol and help flush it from the blood in the body. In a rather controversial study, Dr. Dean Ornish found that a diet rich in soluble fibers actually decreased arteriosclerosis in some patients.

Are You Getting Enough Fiber?: To ascertain if you are one of the nearly 80% of Americans who do not consume enough dietary fiber, get out your calculator. Write down your fiber score for a typical day using the following formula:

	SERVINGS	FIBER (G.)
Fruits, vegetables, Whole grains, nuts	_____ x 2.5 =	_____
Beans, lentils	_____ x 6 =	_____
Refined grains (such as white bread, white rice, regular pasta)	_____ x 1 =	_____
Breakfast cereal (check label for fiber in grams per servings)	_____ x 1 =	_____
Add for daily total grams of fiber		_____

Nutritionists recommend 20 to 30 grams of fiber a day.

Fiber Content of Common Foods

Food	Fiber (g.)	Serving
Vegetables		
Asparagus	.9	4 medium spears
Avocado	2.2	1/2 medium
Broccoli	2.2	1/2 cup
Brussels sprouts	2.3	1/2 cup
Carrots	2.0	1/2 cup
Celery	1.0	1/2 cup
Corn off the cob	4.0	1/2 cup
Corn on the cob	5.9	1 ear
Lettuce	1.0	1 cup
Peas (canned)	4.0	1/2 cup
Peas (dried)	7.9	1/2 cup
Potato (baked with skin)	3.0	1 medium
Spinach (cooked)	5.7	1/2 medium

continued

Food	Fiber (g.)	Serving
Legumes		
Beans	10.0	1/2 cup
(lima, kidney, baked)		
Refried beans	12.0	1 cup
Lentils	8.0	1 cup
Fruits		
Apple with peel	3.5	1 medium
Banana	2.4	1 medium
Grapefruit	1.6	1/2 medium
Nectarine	3.0	1 medium
Orange	2.0	1 medium
Peach	1.8	1 medium
Pear	2.6	1 medium
Strawberries	3.0	1 cup
Kiwi	5.0	1 medium
Cereal and Breads		
Fiber One	14.0	1 cup
100% Bran	13.5	1 cup
All-Bran	10.0	1 cup
Raisin Bran	3.5	1/2 cup
Whole-wheat bread	2.1	1 slice
White, rye, or	.7	1 slice
French bread		
Snacks		
Popcorn (air popped)	4.5	3.5 cups
Sunflower seeds	4.0	1 ounce

Fiber-rich foods are a rare commodity on American shelves. There are indications that dietary deficiency alone could be responsible for our high rates of heart disease and colon cancer.

A psyllium-seed supplement, sprinkled on top of cold cereals or salads, is a safe and healthy way to increase your daily fiber. Other fiber supplements are available in capsule form if you prefer. Psyllium seed (and its husk) is considered the king of fiber sources. But mix it only in cold cereals, yogurts, and juices. When heated, it becomes the consistency of cake batter.

TAKE THIS THOUGHT TO BED WITH YOU

You have made the most important decision in your life, and you've stuck to it!

You have completed more than half the program. You're on the road to success. Take a look back in your logbooks and see the amount of work you've accomplished! Check your calendar. Did you remember to put a gold star on each day you did something extra, exercise-wise, like a walk in the park or a run up a set of stairs?

From now on, there are no excuses. Each day is a new beginning.

Do it! Write it! Be it!

WHAT YOU ATE (If you swallowed it, write it down)

Breakfast: Lunch: Supper:

_____   _____   _____

_____   _____   _____

_____   _____   _____

_____   _____   _____

_____   _____   _____

_____   _____   _____

_____   _____

_____

Snacks:

WHAT YOU DID

Cardiovascular Exercise   Time   Notes

_____   _____   _____

_____   _____   _____

Resistance Exercise   Reps/Sets/Weight   Notes

_____   _____   _____

_____   _____   _____

_____   _____   _____

_____   _____   _____

_____   _____   _____

_____   _____   _____

_____   _____   _____

_____   _____

WHAT YOU THOUGHT

ONLY 13 DAYS TO GO!

DAY 16

BRAIN POWER

When you stop and think about it, today really is the first day of the rest of your life. It's a *now-or-never* day that can hold the key to your continued success.

People don't fail programs because the program doesn't work. People fail when they don't follow through! More than half the battle is won by just stepping up to the plate! You always feel good after doing something good.

Get up, get on the move, and remember you have only 13 more days, so make the most of them (although I highly suspect you'll continue long past our 28-day goal). Today counts.

EATING RIGHT

How have you done with the shopping? Are your shelves filled up with healthy food choices? Have you been concentrating on more protein and low-glycemic carbohydrates in your diet? Have you taken out that pair of shorts or pants to see if they're fitting a bit looser?

If you've been following the program, we should be seeing some bigger changes in the way you look, think, and feel!

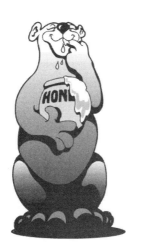
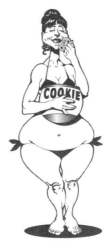

Eat like a bear; look like a pear.
Illustration by Matt Gouig

BREAKFAST

Breakfast on the go: Still too rushed to sit down for breakfast? That's life in the fast lane, so thank goodness for the wide variety in meal replacement bars, shakes, smoothies, and even soups! Remember, never more than two of your three main meals should be replaced by a supplement bar or shake.

Sit-down breakfast: Sauté diced bell pepper, diced onion, and finely diced broccoli crowns in a pan coated with Pam, then add egg substitute, egg whites, or three egg whites with one egg yolk for you yolk-lovers, and scramble them alongside the vegetables. Enjoy the scramble with half a cantaloupe and two slices of rye or pumpernickel bread with almond butter spread. Drink some coffee, tea, or nonfat milk.

When in doubt, think protein. And when you think of protein, think white-meat poultry, lean beef, eggs and egg substitutes, and fish.

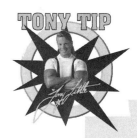

LUNCH

Lunch on the go: Have a meal replacement bar or drink with fresh fruit and plenty of water!

Sit-down lunch: A sandwich made with two slices of sourdough or rye bread, a fist-sized portion of lean meat or a grilled portobello mushroom, a dab of low-fat mayonnaise, a slice of avocado, some lettuce or sprouts, and a slice of tomato sound great.

Have an apple or two apricots for dessert. Drink at least eight ounces of water.

SUPPER

Supper on the go: Heat up a low-sodium soup—lentil, green pea, bean, or barley—and enjoy with rye or pumpernickel bread and lots of water!

Sit-down supper: Choose a fist-sized portion of lean meat, a soy burger, or a Boca burger, grilled. Now go the list of low-glycemic carbohydrates and choose a fist-sized portion of vegetables (yellow, green, or red), a fist-sized portion of carbohydrates, plus one piece of fruit.

Always drink plenty of water with your meals.

WORKOUT

Today it's 30 minutes of cardio. Take your pick, but try to mix it up from week to week. Your body adapts to cardio by becoming more efficient. If you continuously do the same activity, at the same level, your body will not reach its fat-burning zone. Mix it up, and up the ante, and you'll keep getting maximum burn from the time you put in. Get ready to rock!

You can do it!

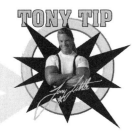

Music makes exercise easier, so crank up some music when you work out. If you're not into the new sounds, then put on something that made you get up and dance when you were younger. Whether it's the Barney song or Led Zeppelin, I want you to get up and rock for your workouts!

CARDIOVASCULAR EXERCISE

Get goin' again. Do the same 30 minutes, but do them at an interval pace. Speed it up for a minute or two every five to six minutes, then cool down. Interval cardio is the most kickin' kind of cardio around! Don't forget the Two-Minute Warning. Time to crank it up! At the end of your cardio workout, just before cool-down, really push yourself to fastest, highest level for two minutes. It's a challenge.

RESISTANCE EXERCISE

Today there's stretching and some more work for your abs. I'd also like you to work on maintaining your sense of balance—something we lose beginning in our thirties. Walk around the house heel-to-toe a few times. Then try standing on one foot for as long as you can. The more you practice these simple moves, the better your balance becomes.

1. Compound crunch (abdominals):

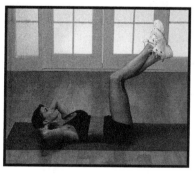 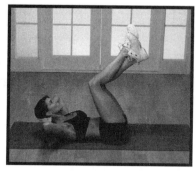

For at home or at the gym. This move works both the upper and lower portions of the abs. This time, perform for ten to 20 repetitions, or until failure (the point at which you just can't do any more!). *Squeeze!*

SET ONE: 10–20 repetitions
SET TWO: 10–20 repetitions
SET THREE: 10–20 repetitions

2. Ab crunch (upper abdominals):

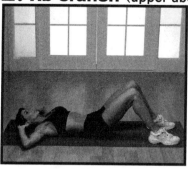 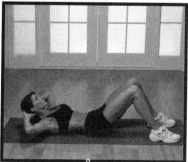

For at home or at the gym. Keep your body as tense as possible and keep these movements slow and precise. Think *squeeze* and technique!

SET ONE: 10–15 repetitions
SET TWO: 10–15 repetitions
SET THREE: 10–15 repetitions

3. Lying back extension (lower back):

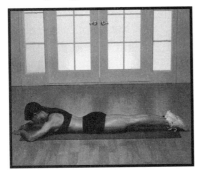 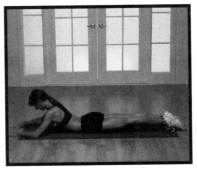

For at home or at the gym. Perform in a smooth, fluid motion. Allow your back to stretch and squeeze as well as flex. This will help keep you from having nagging lower-back pain in the future.

SET ONE: 10–15 repetitions
SET TWO: 10–15 repetitions

HEALTH SMARTS

HIGH CARBOHYDRATES EQUALS HIGH BODY FAT

Low carbphydrates is the buzz of the new millennium. Some zealots even advocate zero carbohydrates!

Come on! Let's learn from our mistakes. We tried zero fat, and all that happened was we got fatter by replacing the fats with carbohydrates. We need all three macronutrients, and don't listen to anyone who says different!

The problem with carbohydrates comes from the type of carbohydrates you eat. There are two types of carbohydrates: simple and complex.

Simple carbohydrates (sugar, corn syrup, fructose, and glucose) are used in baked desserts, drinks, and cereals.

Complex carbohydrates are those contained in vegetables and whole grains. For the most part, these carbohydrates are good and nutritionally beneficial.

Of course, it can't be that simple. When carbohydrates are consumed with other nutrients and additives—such as when you eat ice cream, which contains simple sugars, protein, and preservatives—carbohydrates behave differently in your body than when they are consumed by themselves.

The way scientists have quantified the behavior of sugars is called the glycemic index. This measures the way that food affects the body, including insulin reaction and fat storage. Both are important if you are trying to lose weight and increase your health.

The Fattest Sugar of All?

Recent research has indicated that high-glycemic foods promote fat storage. High-glycemic foods can also stimulate food cravings, and what you crave is more high-glycemic food. Not surprisingly, the Glycemic Index of most fast foods is very high. So not only do the foods taste good, they biologically create their own cravings for more!

Low-glycemic foods do not stimulate fat storage. They get used up as available energy. Some researchers speculate that eating low-glycemic foods may actually help to reduce the size of fat cells, which means you get smaller! Further, eating low-glycemic foods does not contribute to food cravings that can ruin your nutrition plan.

Why Women Crave Chocolate

According to research, women have a particularly difficult time with high-glycemic foods. Estrogen, the primary female hormone that regulates reproductive cycles, is dependent on fat. A woman naturally carries more fat than a man carries. She also stores it more efficiently than a man does. Therefore, most women have a more difficult time than men keeping body fat levels under control.

Nature dictates that women need fat in order to produce estrogen, so biologically women are programmed to crave certain nutrients. At various times of the month serotonin levels fall in women and this stimulates food cravings. Guess what foods increase serotonin levels? Yep, high-glycemic foods.

One of the fastest ways to increase serotonin levels is to ingest fat and simple sugar. What is chocolate? Fat and simple sugar. Bingo! That's why women crave chocolate. Far better would be a snack with olive oil, eggs, or butter in it, followed with fresh fruit. Fat and simple sugar—the healthy way!

TAKE THIS THOUGHT TO BED WITH YOU

Think of a baby's first steps. Before he can learn to walk, the baby must push himself onto his feet and take his first step. If not on the first step, then definitely on the second or third step most babies fall flat on their faces.

But the bewildered child always struggles back up and eventually, step by step, fall by fall, reaches his goal.

You'll make it in much the same way, except that any falling you do will be figurative. Just keep track of any digressions you make from the program—don't forget to record them. Bet you thought I would say it was okay to slip up! Not so! Remember, every bite of food you put in your mouth will affect the outcome of this 28 days. Make it count! Make good choices.

ANOTHER THOUGHT TO TAKE TO BED WITH YOU

Never underestimate the power of the mind. A new hero is born every day—one who faces his or her fear and conquers it. The first step is to believe in yourself, and then reinforce that belief.

When you get up tomorrow, tell yourself, "I can do it!" Go about the day with the confidence of a king or queen who rules their world. Walk straight, tall and proud of who you are and what you do as if your head were in a crown. You were born a winner.

Sleep deeply and rejuvenate for tomorrow.

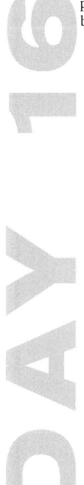

Do it! Write it! Be it!

WHAT YOU ATE (If you swallowed it, write it down)

Breakfast: Lunch: Supper:

_____   _____   _____
_____   _____   _____
_____   _____   _____
_____   _____   _____
_____   _____   _____
_____   _____   _____
_____   _____   _____

Snacks:

WHAT YOU DID

Cardiovascular Exercise   Time   Notes

_____   _____   _____
_____   _____   _____

Ab Exercise   Reps/Sets/Weight   Notes

_____   _____   _____
_____   _____   _____
_____   _____   _____
_____   _____   _____

Other Activities

_____
_____
_____

WHAT YOU THOUGHT

_____

_____

_____

_____

_____

_____

_____

_____

_____

_____

_____

_____

_____

_____

_____

_____

_____

_____

_____

_____

_____

_____

_____

_____

_____

_____

_____

_____

ONLY 12 DAYS TO GO!

DAY 17

BRAIN POWER

Here we go up and over the hump again . . . and I think you are ready for, and deserve, a little R&R. What, you say? Don't go thinking that Tony's going soft on you, but it's always been my belief that for five days out of the week you should treat your body as a temple, and for two as an amusement park.

So let's find some ways to reward ourselves today. With only 12 days left, I think it's about time we have some fun together!

EATING RIGHT

We make dozens of food choices every day of our lives. If a few of those choices are not healthy, other good choices can balance them out. You should look at your food diary from a five- or seven-day perspective. If your total macronutrients are somewhere near the 40-40-20 or 50-30-20 balances I talked about on Day 7, then you're looking good, and I mean that literally.

Yes, it's okay to indulge in some of your favorite foods, once in a while. Just don't go overboard and eat three squares out of the box, Jack. If you know what I mean.

If you're looking for something different, go to the back of the book and check out some of the recipe selections, created in accordance to the 40-40-20 or 50-30-20 plans.

BREAKFAST

Breakfast on the go: Reach for your usual staple of meal replacements, or eat a low-fat, low-sugar yogurt, preferably plain, and a piece of fruit with your coffee or tea and water.

Sit-down breakfast: Have two or three eggs scrambled with low-fat cheddar cheese and three slices of turkey bacon with two slices of rye, sourdough, or pumpernickel bread. Drink a glass of apple juice, or coffee or tea, no sugar, black or with a low-fat cream substitute. Now, are you full and happy? Get yourself off to a really productive day now. Make every second count!

LUNCH

Lunch on the go: How about some Chinese takeout today? Ask for no oil or low oil and no MSG. Stay away from batter-dipped meals and the sweet and sour. Good choices include spring vegetables with bean curd, broccoli and chicken, or black bean chicken. Order steamed rice instead of fried.

Sit-down lunch: Make a sandwich with sourdough, rye, or pumpernickel bread, light mayonnaise, a dab of mustard, and your choice of lean deli meat or tuna. Add lettuce, cheese, and tomato for a high-protein, low-carbohydrate lunch. Have an apple or orange for dessert. Drink at least eight ounces of water.

SUPPER

Supper on the go: Have a big meal replacement shake or smoothie with an extra scoop of protein powder. Enjoy with two pieces of fresh fruit, half a cantaloupe, or apple slices.

Sit-down supper: Grill or broil a fist-sized portion of cube steak (you may substitute tuna steak, salmon, chicken breast, or turkey), and add a fist-sized portion of green beans, lima beans, spinach, or salad with oil and vinegar, fat-free Italian dressing, or balsamic vinegar. Have one sweet or baked potato with light butter or trans-fat-free spread (read the label). Try a bit of A-1 sauce on your potato—it tastes great!

Again, drink plenty of water.

WORKOUT

CARDIOVASCULAR EXERCISE

Feeling sluggish? A cup of tea or coffee can help.

Cardio exercise is not boring. I find it a terrific time to think about the day in front of me and all the opportunities that day brings. I never totally give in to my right-brain thoughts—I still keep my mind on what I'm doing. No leaning on handles, no sleepwalking either. Push it! Always go for it. And you will get it.

Perspiration is what we're seeking here. Even if it's just a tiny glisten on your forehead or neck. You can lose yourself in the music and movement, but stay clear on the concept that you're trying to make your body accomplish a little more each session.

Remember our Perceived Rate of Exertion (PRE)? Well on a scale of 1 to 10, that should be around a 6 or 8 now. Go for 30 minutes and think of the end of your cardio as a two-minute warning in a football game. Make the last two minutes harder and faster, then cool down for five minutes.

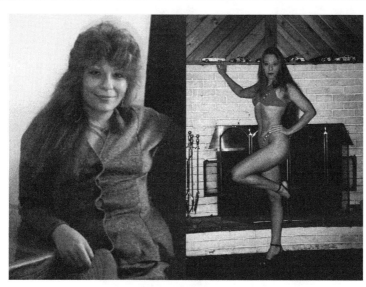

Conceive, believe, achieve!
That's what Jodi Goulding from New York did to lose 30 pounds
of unwanted weight and to feel great!
She's now studying to be a personal trainer.

RESISTANCE EXERCISE

It's back to the weights today! Splash some water in your face and attack this workout. The energy you put in is what burns those calories. You definitely should be feeling the exercise now! Remember, a warm bath at night, plus the stretching and daily cardio helps to keep your muscles limber. If you are extremely sore, cut back until you feel better. Never perform an exercise that hurts you!

We've mixed things up again today! The secret to continued success is to always keep your routines fresh. Exercises done early in a routine are generally done with more effort. Since we trained abs yesterday, I've moved them to the end of this workout today so you can put more work into those super calorie-burning big muscle exercises for the lower body. Burn baby, burn on this one!

1. Full squat (front and back of upper legs and butt):

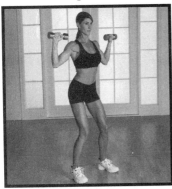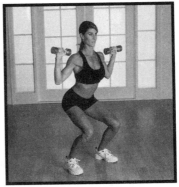

For at home or at the gym. Use five- to 20-pound dumbbells. Slowly lower yourself as if you were about to sit in a chair. Go as far down as you're comfortable, ideally until your thighs are parallel to the floor. As you return, bring your hands back to your hips.

SET ONE: 10–15 repetitions
SET TWO: 10–15 repetitions
SET THREE: 10–15 repetitions

1a. Leg press machine (quads, gluteals):

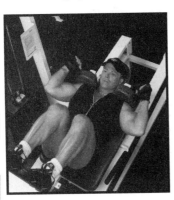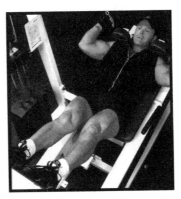

For the gym only. Position the machine so that your knees are bent and you're a little squished at the start. Squeeze your legs out until they are straight, but don't lock the knees. Start to add a little more weight and challenge yourself on this one, but still make the suggested reps. You might be surprised how strong you are and the safety of the machine let's you experiment. Return, under control, to the start. Use weight that is comfortable to perform up to 15 reps with good squeezing exercise form.

SET ONE: 10–15 repetitions
SET TWO: 10–15 repetitions
SET THREE: 10–15 repetitions

2. Stationary lunge (back of upper legs and butt):

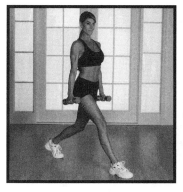 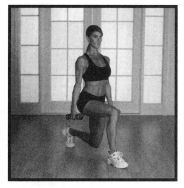

For at home or at the gym. Use your bodyweight or light, five- to 15-pound dumbbells. Perform this lunge by standing upright and taking a large stride forward with your right leg. This is the start position. Let your left knee trail as low as comfortable, but do not touch the floor. Stand back up to the start position, then repeat the lunge. Finish all your reps for one leg before moving to the other leg.

> **SET ONE:** 10–12 repetitions
> **SET TWO:** 10–12 repetitions
> **SET THREE:** 10–12 repetitions

2a. Leg extension (quadriceps):

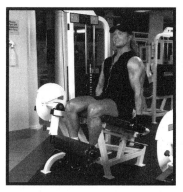 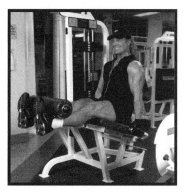

For the gym only. Position yourself in a leg extension machine so the fronts of your ankles are secure behind the pads. Hold onto the side handles. Hold for one second at the peak contraction, then lower the bar. You can go up a little higher in weight as long as you keep your form and reps.

> **SET ONE:** 10–15 repetitions
> **SET TWO:** 10–15 repetitions
> **SET THREE:** 10–15 repetitions

3. Wide-stance squat (legs, inner thighs):

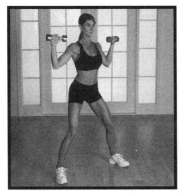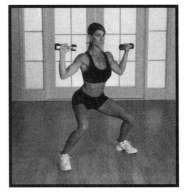

For at home or at the gym. Stand with your feet wider apart than shoulder width, toes pointed out at ten and two o'clock. Hold two light, five- to 15-pound dumbbells at shoulder height. Keep your back straight and eyes up. Squat down as far as comfortable. Then push back up with your legs. Perform this slowly, using a four-count on the way down, a three-count on the way up. *Squeeze* your glutes!

SET ONE: 10–15 repetitions
SET TWO: 10–15 repetitions

3a. Leg press machine (quads, hamstrings, inner thighs):

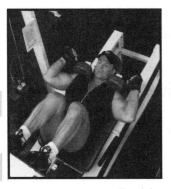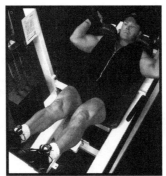

For the gym only. Position yourself so that your feet are as wide apart as possible on the pad, toes pointed out duck-like. This will work your inner thighs. Understand the locking mechanism of the machine before you begin. Push forward to release, then lower the weight as far as comfortable, always under your control. Push back to the start, careful not to lock your knees. Experiment with the heaviest weight you can push and still maintain control of. *Squeeze* your shoulder blades.

SET ONE: 10–15 repetitions
SET TWO: 10–15 repetitions
SET THREE: 10–15 repetitions

4. Back Row with chair (v-taper of back):

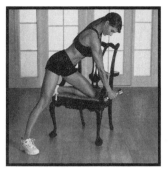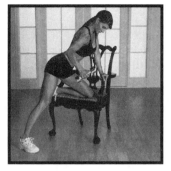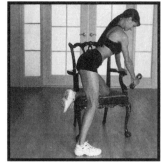

For at home or at the gym. This is a great exercise for strengthening the back. At home, find a sturdy armless chair and kneel on it as shown. In the gym, use a bench. Try and keep your chest almost parallel to the floor and your back straight, balance on the chair with one arm and hold a dumbbell (use a light, 5- to 20-pound dumbbell) at arm's length in the other hand. Keeping your upper body tense, squeeze the dumbbell up to the side of your chest, elbow slightly bent out, then return to arm's length and stretch (but not to the floor).

> **SET ONE:** 10–15 repetitions
> **SET TWO:** 10–15 repetitions
> **SET THREE:** 10–15 repetitions

4a. Lat pulldown (v-taper of back):

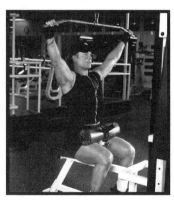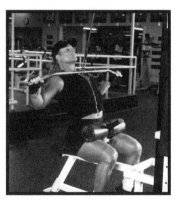

For the gym only. Any wide grip used in a pulling motion exercises the large muscles that run along the sides of the back. Remember to squeeze your shoulder blades together. Position yourself so your knees are secure under the pads. Reach up and take a wide grip on the bar. Squeeze your back muscles as you pull the bar down to your upper chest, arching slightly. Return completely under your control. Use the heaviest weight possible for you to maintain form and complete the reps.

SET ONE: 10–15 repetitions
SET TWO: 10–15 repetitions
SET THREE: 10–15 repetitions

5. Chest crossover (chest):

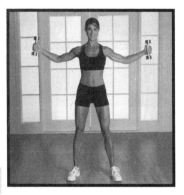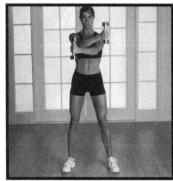

For at home or at the gym. Hold a light, 8- to 15-pound dumbbell in each hand, arms outstretched to your sides. As though you were hugging a barrel, bring the dumbbells together in front of you, one over the other, *squeeze,* and return. Repeat, reversing which arm is on top.

SET ONE: 10–15 repetitions
SET TWO: 10–15 repetitions
SET THREE: 10–15 repetitions

5a. Chest machine or pec deck (chest):

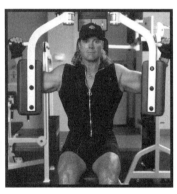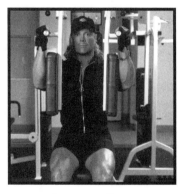

For the gym only. Position the seat so that your forearms are firmly against the pads. With a light grip on the handles squeeze down on your chest muscles and bring the handles together in front of you. Hold for a moment (squeezing) and return to the start. This exercise works the inside of the chest, or the cleavage. Caution: never extend your elbows behind your shoulders.

SET ONE: 10–15 repetitions
SET TWO: 10–15 repetitions
SET THREE: 10–15 repetitions

6. Ab crunch (upper abdominals):

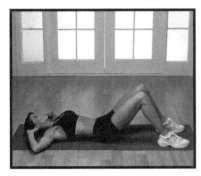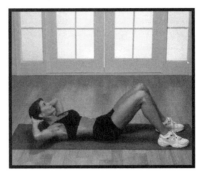

For at home or at the gym. Keep your body as tense as possible and keep these movements slow and precise. Think *squeeze* and technique!

SET ONE: 10–15 repetitions
SET TWO: 10–15 repetitions
SET THREE: 10–15 repetitions

7. Oblique crunch (abdominals):

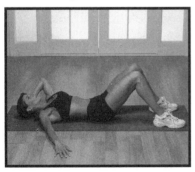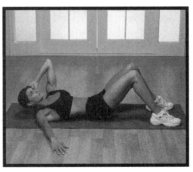

For at home or at the gym. This move works both the abs and the obliques. Knees should be bent and feet flat on the floor. Without pulling your head forward, perform an ab crunch with your chin up, pulling your left elbow and shoulder toward your right knee. Alternate with your right elbow and shoulder pulling toward your left knee.

SET ONE: 10–15 repetitions
SET TWO: 10–15 repetitions
SET THREE: 10–15 repetitions

You are becoming a true lifter! And probably getting a little sore. Don't worry, that's a sign that you're doing everything right. Before you finish off for the day, perform some light stretching. (See page 301.)

HEALTH SMARTS

THE FISHY FACTS ON SEAFOOD

When God put man and woman on earth with the intention that they should live happily ever after, I believe He set in motion our society's penchant for contradicting ourselves. While candidates running for office easily hold a record for canceling out what they say from one speech to the next, nutritionists and others in the food and supplement fields must be in a solid second place. Consider some of the things we've been told in just the last ten years: meat should be served with every meal; limit meat to the middle of the food pyramid; eat lots of dairy; avoid dairy; eat pasta; don't eat pasta; fat-free is good; fat-free makes you fat (this is only true when you forget portion size and overeat the fat-free foods).

Arrgghh! It's enough to drive anyone nuts. Most of the time it's just irritating prattle, but once in a while, the message being sent out is downright unhealthy. One very healthy food source that is unjustly maligned is seafood.

I live near (and swim, boat, and fish in) the gulf waters off the coast of Florida. In all my years here I can tell you that I've never seen an obese-looking fish that wasn't pregnant. Fish do contain fat, but it comes in the form of oils. The type of fat in fish oil is usually very low in saturated fat—the bad fat—and often very high in polyunsaturated fatty acids, known as omega-3s. These healthy oils have anti-clotting properties and thus may be protective against heart attacks and high blood pressure.

Therefore, contrary to what some people may tell you, seafood is not a bad food to consume, and only a few types are high enough in fat to set off the alarm of even a strict dieter's calorie counter. (Most seafood has less fat than a skinless chicken breast.)

Americans have traditionally favored meat over seafood. Americans also have alarming rates of cancer and heart disease, higher even than people living in countries where the standard diet includes fats from rich, creamy sauces. Lean red meat once or twice a week is okay. But the good news is that since the early 1980s annual consumption of fish and shellfish has risen by more than 25%.

Are Today's Fish Contaminated?

Sure, fish in the new millennium are likely to have contaminants that simply weren't present in the 1900s. So does new millennium air, but we don't stop breathing, do we?

Many people believe that bottom-dwelling fish and seafood, such as catfish and flounder as well as shrimp, crab, and lobster, feed mainly off waste. Actually, they eat whatever swims or floats by them, their taste buds having less discrimination than the family dog's. They have very efficient systems and are able to convert even dead organic matter into proteins, fats, and carbohydrates. They are *not* necessarily more likely to be contaminated than other fish.

Seafood is among the most perishable food we consume. You should eat it within 48 hours of it being caught or thawed. It should also come from a reputable fish handler and it is always good to know its source.

Always cook seafood thoroughly and check for freshness. If the cat turns away at the smell of your raw fish, I'd toss it in the dumpster. But under ordinary circumstances, fish is safe when cooked and stored properly.

To be safe, eat fish and shellfish in reasonable amounts, not more than three times a week. Before you eat freshwater fish caught locally, check with the local health department to make sure the waters are safe.

Fish are your most nutritious source of protein. Even if you have plenty of protein in your diet, seafood is loaded with other valuable and essential nutrients. If, like many Americans, you simply don't like seafood, you should consider using a fish oil supplement.

TAKE THIS THOUGHT TO BED WITH YOU

The health industry is filled with many contradictions. No one program or diet will work for everyone. Each of us is different—chemically, emotionally, and physically. That's why there are so many programs and diets floating around out there.

But this One-on-One program leaves you room for choice so you can customize this program to your lifestyle, schedule, and needs.

A healthy diet feels good. Too many sweets, and too much of any food (nutritious or not) leaves us feeling bloated and uncomfortable. When you eat, and especially right after you eat, think about the way you feel.

If you eat to feel healthy and energized, then you're eating healthy. It's as simple as that. If you eat healthy, you look and feel healthy. This is a fact, Jack! (Or Jill!)

Do it! Write it! Be it!

WHAT YOU ATE (If you swallowed it, write it down)

Breakfast: Lunch: Supper:

_____   _____   _____
_____   _____   _____
_____   _____   _____
_____   _____   _____
_____   _____   _____
_____   _____   _____
_____   _____   _____
_____   _____   _____

Snacks:

WHAT YOU DID

Cardiovascular Exercise   Time   Notes

_____   _____   _____
_____   _____   _____

Resistance Exercise   Reps/Sets/Weight   Notes

_____   _____   _____
_____   _____   _____
_____   _____   _____
_____   _____   _____
_____   _____   _____
_____   _____   _____
_____   _____   _____
_____   _____   _____

WHAT YOU THOUGHT

ONLY 11 DAYS TO GO!

DAY 18

BRAIN POWER

The finish line is within sight—and it feels like we just started! Are you beginning to see how the simple changes you've made to your life can change your life?

Get up today and be a little selfish. Take a few extra moments to make sure you're eating healthy. Take a few extra minutes to get the exercise you need. Then see if you can make a new friend today. After all, at the rate you're going you'll be around for a long time to come, so it's nice to have all the friends you can.

EATING RIGHT

How about taking a friend to lunch or dinner today? Show off your new skills at making healthy menu choices, asking for dressings on the side, asking for broiled or grilled instead of fried, and choosing lean protein sources.

Chances are that your friend will follow suit or make similar healthy choices.

> **It's a fact:** Good health is contagious; spread it around!

BREAKFAST

Breakfast on the go: Reach for a balanced high-protein, low-carbohydrate meal replacement. For in-between hunger attacks, how about a fist-sized portion of lean deli meat or a hard-boiled egg.

Sit-down breakfast: Time for another south-of-the-border burrito for the extra thermogenic properties that help burn calories! Wrap some sautéed fresh vegetables with scrambled eggs or tofu in a reduced-fat tortilla. Add salsa and hot peppers to taste. Enjoy with a cup of coffee or tea, and one slice of whole-grain, rye, or pumpernickel bread.

Record what you eat, what you do, and what you think!

LUNCH

Lunch on the go: Have soup and salad at a deli or sandwich bar that makes home-made soups. Avoid cream-based soups in favor of broth-based soups. Use no more than two tablespoons of dressing on your salad. Drink plenty of water.

Sit-down lunch: Make it a soup-and-salad day! Seek out bean, lentil, or pea soup. Make it from scratch, a soup starter, or out of the can. Always seek out low-sodium canned soups such as Healthy Choice. Use low-fat or nonfat dressing, and not more than two tablespoons on your green and leafy salad. Have fruit for dessert and drink at least eight ounces of water.

SUPPER

Supper on the go: Choose a meal replacement shake or smoothie with fresh fruit. Have a handful of raw mixed nuts and a low-fat, low-sugar yogurt. Drink lots of water and snack on celery and carrot sticks.

Sit-down supper: Have you had your fish today? Try a salmon steak, mahi-mahi, sole, or swordfish, broiled in the oven or on a George Foreman grill. Have this with a cup of wild rice and a medley of mixed green, orange, and yellow veggies (broccoli, carrots, yellow peppers) with mushrooms, lightly stir-fried in a tablespoon of olive oil.

Always drink plenty of water with your meals. A diet soda is in order tonight if you prefer.

WORKOUT

We're back to hitting the cardio and abs again. Have you established a training time for both your cardio and your resistance? Consistent times make it easier for you to form a habit, and harder for you to break from the assigned course.

Your workout schedule will stay consistent until you achieve your goal weight.

At that point, you can cut back your cardio to three to four days a week. But for now, your program is this:

MONDAY: Cardio and resistance
TUESDAY: Cardio and abs
WEDNESDAY: Cardio and resistance
THURSDAY: Cardio and abs
FRIDAY: Cardio and resistance
SATURDAY: Active rest/cardio (your last week will have abs as well)
SUNDAY: Off/active rest

CARDIOVASCULAR EXERCISE

Pick your form of cardio: walking, marching, stair climbing, gliding, exercising on the treadmill, cycling, or low-impact aerobic dancing. Go for the burn, go for the interval, and go for a "bonus" five minutes today. That's 35 minutes of continuous, nonstop, fat-burning exercise! Remember, cardio is best for fat burning in the morning.

1. Reverse crunch (lower abdominals):

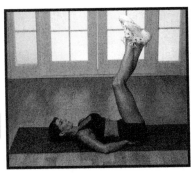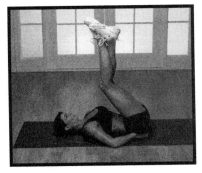

For at home or at the gym. Think technique! Don't let that lower back come too far off the ground, and breathe out as you bear down on the lower abs.

SET ONE: 10–15 repetitions
SET TWO: 10–15 repetitions
SET THREE: 10–15 repetitions

2. Compound crunch (abdominals):

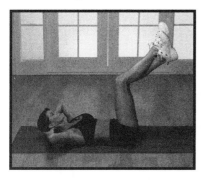 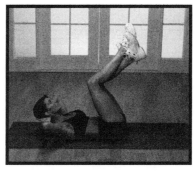

For at home or at the gym. This move works both the upper and lower portions of the abs. Again, perform these for ten to 20 repetitions, or until failure (the point at which you just can't do any more).

SET ONE: 10–20 repetitions
SET TWO: 10–20 repetitions
SET THREE: 10–20 repetitions

Finish off with a stretch for the lower back.

> ### Don't forget to record what you eat, what you do, and what you think.

HEALTH SMARTS

WHICH IS MORE IMPORTANT: EXERCISE OR DIET?

While many people wait to choose one over the other, my initial reaction to this question was similar to how I might feel if I had to choose between my two kids. Sorry, I don't go there, can't do that. They both enrich my life. Like my kids, diet and exercise each have unique qualities, and although different, each is equally valid, essential, and worthy.

If you're wondering which is more important, you might be a person unaccustomed to regular exercise and unmotivated to make drastic changes in your diet. You are most likely looking for an easy way out. Perhaps the better question is where do you start on a program toward better health—with diet or exercise? Eventually, both must be employed; but for the time being let's start out slow.

Diet

You make food choices every day. Even if someone else is doing the shopping and putting the food on the table, you decide on your portions and preferences. You are already controlling your diet, and that's all "dieting" is. Throw out the notion that you are going to have to deny yourself some of life's greatest pleasures. Instead, educate yourself about foods and make better choices that give your body its optimum nutrition, as well as great taste.

Remember, the Clean Plate Club does not exist! There is no need to eat everything on your plate. You cannot put your leftovers in an envelope to send away to feed a starving child. Stop eating when you are satisfied.

One thing for certain is that saturated fat is not a good thing. It's contained in fatty meats and full-fat dairy products. But you've already learned that all fat is not bad. You don't need to stop eating cheese and meat. You just need to begin to limit some of these foods or switch to low-fat varieties.

Exercise

As you've discovered, you don't have to pull on a pair of spandex shorts and join an expensive health club to get exercise. The entire routine in this program can be done at home. The best type of exercise for weight loss is one that involves cardio up to seven days a week, and resistance training for up to four days a week.

Studies have shown that people who lose weight through diet alone are much more likely to gain the weight back than people who use a combination of diet and exercise. Diet alone can actually destroy lean muscle mass, and we all know muscle requires more calories for maintenance than other tissue so it's very beneficial in keeping the weight off, with minimum changes to diet.

It is impossible to say that exercise or diet is better than the other. They both work together for our good health.

The challenge is that exercise takes time. While your strength gains may come quickly, it can take months to build a pound of lean muscle mass. But once you build it, that lean muscle tissue continues to burn calories throughout the day. A pound of fat just sits there!

In the beginning, changes to your diet will have the most obvious effect on your bodyweight and proportions. But in the long term, exercise will keep your weight under control, allow you to eat more freely, and give you the tone and energy levels you seek.

Resistance exercise is great for anti-aging because it helps reverse and slow down the loss of muscle due to the natural aging process. Resistance exercise helps keep you young.

TAKE THIS THOUGHT TO BED WITH YOU

Eighteen days gone and just ten more to go. But, like graduating from school, our goal of feeling better, looking better will only be reached when all the studying and exams are over. We're still learning what our bodies need in the way of fuel and exercise to prepare us for the tests that life will bring.

Think about how far you want to take this fitness quest. We've accomplished a lot, and there's still more down the road. How much are you willing to put in?

The more energy you put in, the more you get out. Every success story contains this simple truth: What you give is what you get.

You've had a big day, so you need a good night's rest. Get up tomorrow morning and kick butt! But make sure it's your own.

DAY 18

Do it! Write it! Be it!

WHAT YOU ATE (If you swallowed it, write it down)

Breakfast: Lunch: Supper:

_____   _____   _____
_____   _____   _____
_____   _____   _____
_____   _____   _____
_____   _____   _____
_____   _____   _____
_____   _____   _____
_____   _____   _____

Snacks:

WHAT YOU DID

Cardiovascular Exercise   Time   Notes

_____   _____   _____

Ab Exercise   Reps/Sets/Weight   Notes

_____   _____   _____
_____   _____   _____
_____   _____   _____
_____   _____   _____

Other Activities

_____
_____

Stretches

_____

WHAT YOU THOUGHT

_____
_____
_____
_____
_____
_____
_____
_____
_____
_____
_____
_____
_____
_____
_____
_____
_____
_____
_____
_____
_____
_____
_____
_____
_____
_____
_____
_____
_____

ONLY 10 DAYS TO GO!

DAY 19

BRAIN POWER

You're still with me! Congratulations! It's a fact that many people start an exercise program and never make it through week three. The first week they're gung-ho. The second week they're so-so, and by the end of the third, they're oh no! Gone! The fact you've made it this far tells me you can make it all the way—and beyond.

Go for it! It's a new day and a new beginning.

EATING RIGHT

This is getting to be a habit, isn't it? Like second nature? That's the way it's supposed to be. And are you fitting into those tight pants that refused to zip up just three weeks ago? Yeah, that's what I thought! Good job!

BREAKFAST

Breakfast on the go: Have Kashi brand high-fiber cereal with nonfat milk and a piece of fruit or a meal replacement bar or drink.

Sit-down breakfast: Start with a scoop of protein powder mixed with low-fat yogurt, preferably plain, berries, fruits and nuts. Add two slices of whole-grain or rye bread with butter, almond butter, or a spread that does not contain trans fat. Or, have a traditional breakfast of eggs with toast and fruit. For a drink, have a cup of coffee or tea, no sugar, black or with a low-fat cream substitute.

LUNCH

Lunch on the go: Enjoy a deli-made tuna salad with lots of greens and not more than two tablespoons of dressing. Many delis now prepare their tuna with low-fat mayonnaise.

Sit-down lunch: Prepare one fist-sized lean hamburger patty, turkey patty or low-fat veggie burger cooked on a George Foreman grill or fried with Pam. (For flavor, dip in A-1 sauce or ketchup.) On the side have a slice of avocado, cottage cheese, and warm black or kidney beans.

Have an apple or orange for dessert. Drink at least eight ounces of water.

SUPPER

Supper on the go: Have a meal replacement high-protein shake with extra fresh fruit and a handful of unsalted walnuts and almonds, plus lots of water.

Sit-down supper: Grill or bake your choice of flank steak, sole, or tofu scramble or patties. Add a fist-sized portion of a green vegetable, or salad with oil and vinegar, fat-free Italian dressing, or balsamic vinegar. Enjoy one cup of rice; wild is preferred, but brown or white will do. Go easy on the soy sauce. And don't ever, ever forget to drink plenty of water.

WORKOUT

Feeling muscles you never knew you had before? During today's workout try to really get in touch with your muscles. If you have a mirror, perform the exercises in front of it and really watch the muscle work. Direct 100% of your mental energy right to that muscle group.

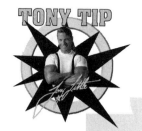

Individuals who train with mental concentration increase the effectiveness of their exercise time. Time is the one commodity that cannot be replaced. We need to pack the most into the limited time we have! The more you do in the shortest time gives you the most results.

CARDIOVASCULAR EXERCISE

Here we go again. Invest 35 minutes of your time. Remember to work at a PRE (Perceived Rate of Exertion) of 7 to 8. You should sweat.

RESISTANCE EXERCISE

Okay, time to muster up some energy for one more killer calorie-burning workout—then you'll have two days of rest. You can do it; it's your last workout of the week!

I took out the ab exercises today so you can really put in a calorie-burning, lean muscle-building workout!

Challenge yourself by increasing resistance on every exercise, but not so much that you have to sacrifice the squeeze technique.

1. Full squat (front and back of upper legs and butt):

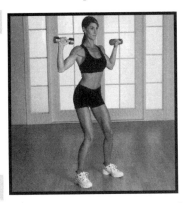 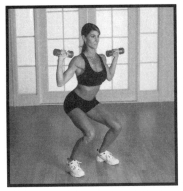

For at home or at the gym. Stand with your feet shoulder-width apart. Hold 5- to 20-pound dumbbells (as shown). Now slowly lower yourself as if you were about to sit in a chair. At the same time bring your arms out in front of you for balance. Go as far down as you're comfortable with, ideally until your thighs are parallel to the floor.

SET ONE: 10–15 repetitions
SET TWO: 10–15 repetitions
SET THREE: 10–15 repetitions

1a. Leg press (front upper legs and butt):

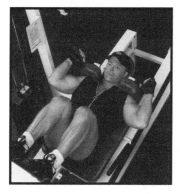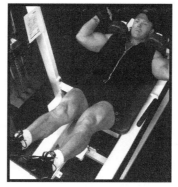

For the gym only. Position the machine so that your knees are bent and you're a little squished at the start. Push your legs and squeeze out until they are straight, but don't lock the knees. Then return, under control, to the start. Machines vary, so experiment with the poundage—you might be a lot stronger on this than you think!

> **SET ONE:** 10–15 repetitions
> **SET TWO:** 10–15 repetitions
> **SET THREE:** 10–15 repetitions

2. Walking lunge (hamstrings, gluteals):

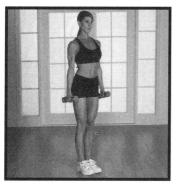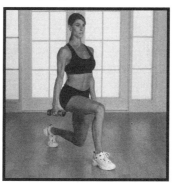

For at home or at the gym. Here's a new one! Use your own bodyweight or light, 5- to 10-pound dumbbells. Stand upright and take a large stride forward with your right leg. Let your left knee trail as low as comfortable, but do not touch the floor. Now begin to stand upright and take another stride with your left leg—as if you are walking. Count each step as one rep and strive for the recommended reps or until failure. Remember to squeeze up on each repetition.

> **SET ONE:** 20–25 repetitions
> **SET TWO:** 20–25 repetitions
> **SET THREE:** 20–25 repetitions

DAY 19

2a. Leg extension (quadriceps):

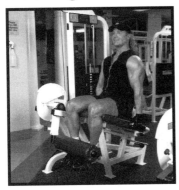 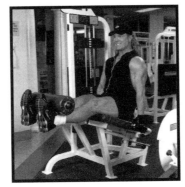

For the gym only. Position yourself in a leg extension machine so the fronts of your ankles are secure behind the pads. Hold onto the side handles. Squeeze your quads as you extend your legs straight out in front of you. Hold for one second at the peak contraction, then lower the bar.

> **SET ONE:** 10–15 repetitions
> **SET TWO:** 10–15 repetitions
> **SET THREE:** 10–15 repetitions

3. Wide-stance squat (legs, hamstrings, inner thighs):

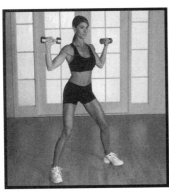 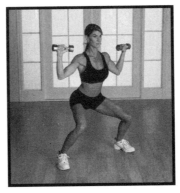

For at home or at the gym. With 8- to 20-pound dumbbells held (as shown), stand with your feet wider apart than shoulder width and your toes pointed out at ten and two o'clock. If you wish, you may rest the ends of the dumbbells on your shoulders. Keep your back straight and eyes up and squat down as far as comfortable. Then push back up with your legs. Perform this slowly, using a four-count on the way down and a three-count on the way up. *Squeeze* your glutes!

> **SET ONE:** 10–15 repetitions
> **SET TWO:** 10–15 repetitions
> **SET THREE:** 10–15 repetitions

DAY 19

4. Modified push-up or push-up (chest):

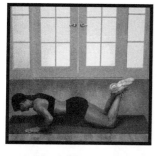 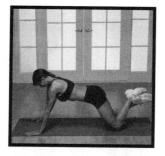

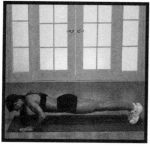 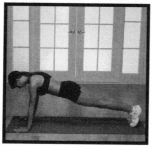

For at home or at the gym. You may perform this according to your conditioning. The easiest way is to perform it leaning against a table-high object. A more difficult push-up may be done lying flat on the floor and pushing up from your knees (as shown). The hardest form of push-up is lying flat on your stomach and pushing your entire body up from the floor while only your hands and toes are touching the floor. In all the different variations, your hands should be positioned just outside your shoulders, arms slightly bent out, elbows in line with your shoulders, back straight, and your neck in a neutral position. Lower down to the point just before your chest touches the floor and then squeeze your chest muscles as you raise up, repeat.

SET ONE: 10–15 repetitions
SET TWO: 10–15 repetitions
SET THREE: 10–15 repetitions

DAY 19

4a. Chest press machine (chest):

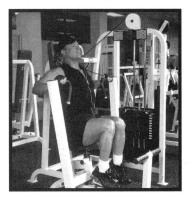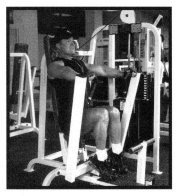

For at the gym only. With your feet firmly on the pad, tense your upper body, particularly your chest, and push the weight directly in front of you. Hold for one-half second at the peak contraction, then return under control. Check your log and increase your weight this time.

SET ONE: 10–15 repetitions
SET TWO: 10–15 repetitions
SET THREE: 10–15 repetitions

5. Back Row with chair (v-taper of back):

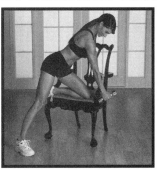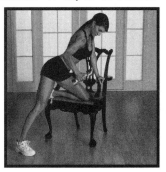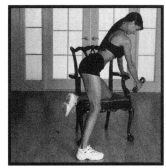

For at home or at the gym. This is a great exercise for strengthening the back. At home, find a sturdy armless chair and kneel on it as shown. In the gym, use a bench. Try and keep your chest almost parallel to the floor and your back straight, balance on the chair with one arm and hold a dumbbell (use a light, 5- to 20-pound dumbbell) at arm's length in the other hand. Keeping your upper body tense, squeeze the dumbbell up to the side of your chest, elbow slightly bent out, then return to arm's length and stretch (but not to the floor).

SET ONE: 10–15 repetitions

SET TWO: 10–15 repetitions
SET THREE: 10–15 repetitions

5a. Back row machine (back):

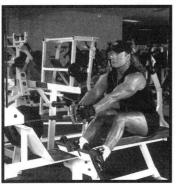 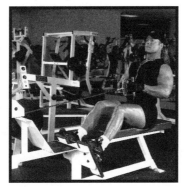

For the gym only. Grab the close-grip handles on a rowing machine with a 45-degree back, then push back with your legs until there is tension on the cable. From this position, pull the handles close to your body and squeeze your shoulder blades at the peak of the movement. Return to the original position and stretch. Try extra weight on the first set; if this is too heavy, drop back for sets two and three.

SET ONE: 10–15 repetitions
SET TWO: 10–15 repetitions
SET THREE: 10–15 repetitions

6. Shoulder press (shoulders):

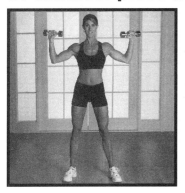 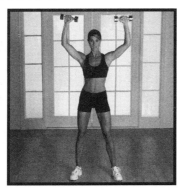

For at home or at the gym. This is a basic shoulder exercise. With knees slightly bent, stand with your feet shoulder-width apart. Holding a light, 5- to 15-pound dumbbell in each hand, bring them up to shoulder height, palms facing away from your body. In a slight arc, lift the dumbbells simultaneously up above your head. Return to the original position.

SET ONE: 10–15 repetitions
SET TWO: 10–15 repetitions
SET THREE: 10–15 repetitions

6a. Seated shoulder press (shoulders):

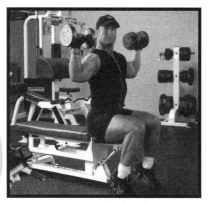 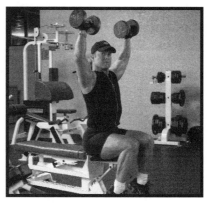

For the gym only. Sit on the end of a bench with dumbbells in both hands. Begin with the dumbbells held as shown. Tensing your arms, shoulders, and torso, slowly bring the dumbbells up in an arc to arms' length (as shown). Return to the original position. Go heavy, but not so heavy you sacrifice form.

SET ONE: 10–15 repetitions
SET TWO: 10–15 repetitions
SET THREE: 10–15 repetitions

7. Concentration curl (biceps):

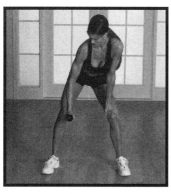 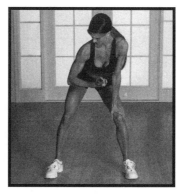

For at home or at the gym. Rest one arm on your knee. With an 8- to 20-pound dumbbell in the other hand, slowly curl it up toward your chest. Really squeeze throughout the movement up, and down. Perform all reps for one arm before moving to the other arm.

SET ONE: 10–15 repetitions
SET TWO: 10–15 repetitions
SET THREE: 10–15 repetitions

7a. Arm curl machine or preacher bench (biceps):

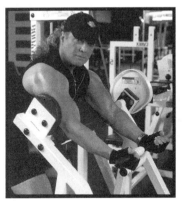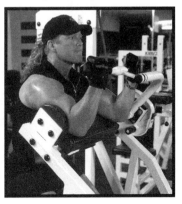

For the gym only. Adjust the set so you can hold the handles at arms' length. Squeezing hard on your biceps, curl the handles up as high as possible. Hold and really squeeze for the peak contraction, then return slowly. Don't use heavy weight.

SET ONE: 10–15 repetitions
SET TWO: 10–15 repetitions
SET THREE: 10–15 repetitions

8. Triceps extension (back of upper arms):

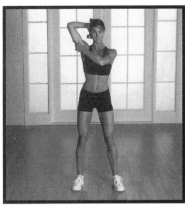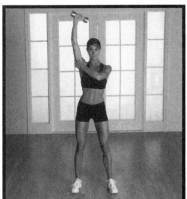

For at home or at the gym. Begin with a 5- to 20-pound dumbbell as shown. Keeping your upper arm in place, lower the weight as far as comfortable behind your head. Now bring the dumbbell back to arm's length as shown. Repeat for the other arm.

SET ONE: 10–12 repetitions
SET TWO: 10–12 repetitions
SET THREE: 10–12 repetitions

8a. Seated triceps pushdown on machine
(back of upper arms):

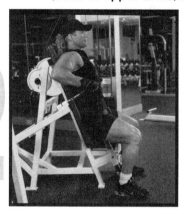 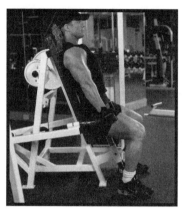

For the gym only. Sit in a triceps pushdown machine and grab both handles. Your feet should be solid on the floor. Squeezing your triceps, press the handles down to arms' length. As you return, keep tension on the triceps.

SET ONE: 10–12 repetitions
SET TWO: 10–12 repetitions
SET THREE: 10–12 repetitions

Finish off with some light stretching. Walking around will loosen up those leg muscles!

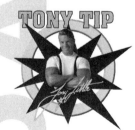

Move it with mental muscle! Put some brains behind the brawn! Concentrate and think technique! You are what you think you are! Use mind and muscle!

HEALTH SMARTS

UNSCRAMBLING THE EGG ISSUE

In the past, eggs have gotten a really bad rap, but new studies have been showing that eggs are actually a pretty perfect food. It's no wonder they've won the starring roles on our breakfast tables! They are an inexpensive source of high protein and vitamins, and if you eat a healthy diet with plenty of fiber, eggs are not only nutritious but versatile as well. (Eggs on their own have no fiber.)

How Healthy Are Eggs?

The argument some nutritionists have with eggs lies in the amount of saturated fat contained in one large egg: nearly five grams! Higher amounts of saturated fat can lead to a higher amount of cholesterol buildup in your circulatory system, especially in the arteries, which can cause heart disease or even a heart attack.

One solution is to eat the egg whites and not the yolks. Egg whites contain all the rich protein that you want without the cholesterol and the calories. An egg white scramble with cottage cheese tastes like whole eggs; of course, your scramble is white, not yellow. Another solution is to use egg substitutes. And everyone agrees that eggs should be limited to six to ten a week.

Always cook eggs. Raw eggs can carry contaminants, but cooking eliminates this.

Mix It Up

Egg protein is an essential part of my diet and should be in yours as well. If you are concerned about the fat and cholesterol, use egg substitutes. If you do not know if you should be concerned, call your doctor.

Due to the high quality of protein in eggs, there are many egg- and protein-based meal replacement drinks, shakes, and bars to choose from. While they may not be the same as poached eggs and bacon, a shake mixed up with fresh fruit and ice can be a delicious and nutritious way to start the day!

TAKE THIS THOUGHT TO BED WITH YOU

Go back to Day 1 and read through all your logbooks tonight. Think of what you've accomplished and how far you've come in conditioning, changing your proportions, weight lost, and a healthier, happier mental attitude. Write down some of those thoughts in the logbook. Then when you go to sleep, think about what else you can do to make your life healthier and happier.

Sweet dreams. No screams. Good night!

Do it! Write it! Be it!

WHAT YOU ATE (If you swallowed it, write it down)

Breakfast: Lunch: Supper:

_____   _____   _____
_____   _____   _____
_____   _____   _____
_____   _____   _____
_____   _____   _____
_____   _____   _____
_____   _____   _____
_____   _____   _____

Snacks:

WHAT YOU DID

Cardiovascular Exercise   Time   Notes

_____   _____   _____
_____   _____   _____

Resistance Exercise   Reps/Sets/Weight   Notes

_____   _____   _____
_____   _____   _____
_____   _____   _____
_____   _____   _____
_____   _____   _____
_____   _____   _____
_____   _____   _____
_____   _____   _____

WHAT YOU THOUGHT

ONLY 9 DAYS TO GO!

DAY 20

Many Europeans say that Americans don't know how to vacation or to just plain "chill." Our gotta-have-it-now attitude is what has made fast food so popular here. If we stopped to smell the roses—and got our noses out of our laptops—we'd most likely find a world of stimulating activity that excites us mentally and physically. I think we'd also learn to relax.

The Chinese refer to a healthy balance in life as the ying and yang. An active lifestyle requires an equal amount of time for relaxation, rest, and sleep. For most of us, the weekends are that time. Make sure to make good use of them. Once in a while, it's okay just to do nothing.

EATING RIGHT

Now you're getting the hang of healthy eating. If you're the chef in the house, you might look up one of your favorite recipes and figure out how to cut out the butter (replace with applesauce), lower the sugar (replace with crushed fruit cocktail), and reduce fat (use olive oil, canola oil, or a trans-fat-free spread and lean cuts of meat). Be creative. It's easy to come up with healthy versions of your favorite foods!

BREAKFAST

Breakfast on the go: Are your cupboards full of meal replacements you can choose from when you're in a hurry? If not, stock up! This morning, grab a meal replacement bar or drink and a piece of fruit, then rush out the door with your water bottle in hand!

Sit-down breakfast: Have one whole-wheat bagel with reduced-fat cream cheese, each side topped with lox, sardines, smoked salmon, or a slice of deli meat if you like. Enjoy a cup of coffee or tea, no sugar, black or with a low-fat cream substitute, and a piece of fresh, in-season fruit.

LUNCH

Lunch on the go: It's tough to go wrong with salads. Get a chunky chicken salad, fajita salad (without sour cream), chef's salad, or Cobb salad (without the bacon and blue cheese). Keep dressings on the side and limit them to no more than two tablespoons. Add olives, shredded cheese, bacon bits, and/or sunflower seeds for extra flavor.

Sit-down lunch: Enjoy a hearty bowl of lentil, barley, or vegetable soup with rye or pumpernickel bread. Have a slice of cheese and fresh fruit for dessert. And drink lots of water!

SUPPER

Supper on the go: Grab a meal replacement shake or smoothie. Make it yourself with fresh fruit and additional low-fat yogurt, preferably plain, and/or protein. Drink lots of water.

Sit-down supper: Choose a lean protein source, then check the list of low-glycemic carbohydrates for vegetables and a carbohydrate. Fix proper proportions for yourself and enjoy. Or, take yourself out to a restaurant and request selections from your list.

Sorbet or fruit and cheese for dessert are great. Always drink plenty of water with your meals.

WORKOUT

Today's another day of active rest/cardio. Can you think of something relaxing to do? How about a long walk through a public garden, museum, or aquarium? How about finding an elderly friend and taking them for a little walk and talk in the park, then volunteering to do a couple of chores around their house? Don't forget to put a gold star on your calendar for every day you get out and do a little bit more than usual, or do something for someone else. One way or the other, get in 30 minutes of continuous movement today.

We're skipping resistance today, but I'd like you to learn a new move that comes from the Chinese. It's a simple hip circle, and can be done anywhere, anytime, for as long as you like. It may be why the Chinese have less back pain than we stiff Americans. Loosen up and give it a try.

1. Side twist (trunk, low back):

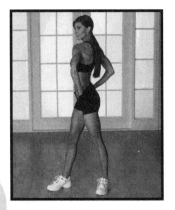 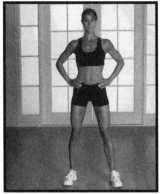 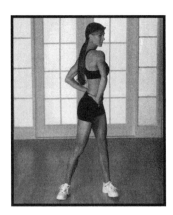

For at home or at the gym. This is a wonderful exercise for the lower back. Keep your shoulders still, and use the muscles below your waist to swivel or twist your hips in a fluid motion, clockwise. After you've finished the prescribed reps, repeat counter-clockwise. Standing in front of a mirror helps you keep your shoulders straight.

SET ONE: 10–20 repetitions each direction
SET TWO: 10–20 repetitions each direction

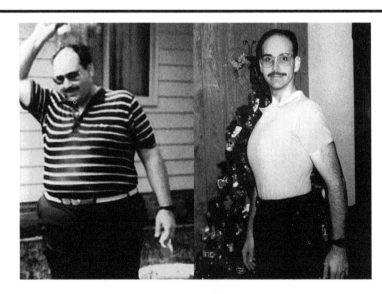

Never say never. Paul Avallone from Ohio lost 153 pounds using Tony's techniques and videos to change his life! You can do it too! He is truly an inspiration.

HEALTH SMARTS

IS RED MEAT EVIL?

For the past couple of decades red meat has come under fire from just about every health-food advocate group, but it really is a staple of the American diet.

Most Americans eat meat at almost every meal. Yet consumption of beef dropped significantly in the early 1990s due to concern over its high saturated fat and cholesterol content. As people have grown weary of the no-fat diet, beef consumption has been on the rise again.

The good news is that the beef you eat today contains about 27% less fat than it did 20 years ago. This fancy feat has come about by selective breeding for leaner animals, the slaughter of them at a younger age, and the trimming away of excess fat from the cuts. Red meat in your diet two or three times a week is fine, but you must watch the cuts you eat.

All beef contains saturated fat, and even the leanest cuts are still higher in fat than broiled fish or skinless chicken. Beef is graded by government inspectors. The highest grade—prime—is the fattiest, followed by choice. Select grades have the least marbling and fat content, although they may not be as juicy and flavorful as the higher grades. Only about 44% of beef is graded; I suggest you look for select grades.

Your next guideline is cut. Brisket, chuck, rib, and ground beef are among the fattiest. Flank, round, and sirloin are leaner. Here are some comparisons of cuts of beef:

FATTIEST CUTS	PERCENTAGE OF FAT BY WEIGHT
Blade Roast, Prime	21
Prime Rib	19
Lean Ground Beef	18
Short Ribs	18
Top Loin, Choice	14
Flank, Choice	13
Sirloin, Prime	12
Rib Eye, Choice	12

Leanest Cuts	Percentage of Fat by Weight
Eye of Round, Choice	6
Bottom Round, Select	5
Tip Round, Select	5
Buffalo	5
Top Round, Select	4
Eye of Round, Select	4

Beef Bits

- Beef liver is loaded with vitamins and minerals; however, just 3.5 ounces provides 369 milligrams of cholesterol, more than the recommended maximum daily allowance.
- Veal is leaner than beef.
- Beef jerky tends to be very high in sodium, and some types can have up to 12 grams of fat per ounce.
- Ground meats are not subject to the same labeling laws pertaining to fat content as other cuts of meat.

When shopping for ground beef, beware of labels that say "10% fat," or conversely, "90% lean." Due to a loophole in meat labeling, these numbers refer to the percentage of fat by weight, not the percentage of calories from fat. In reality, the 10% ground beef still derives half its calories from fat. The 15% gets 61% of its calories from fat and the 25% gets a whopping 75% of its calories from fat!

Fast-food burgers are not healthy. Period. I won't go into the cooking process and other factors that make fast-food burgers a slow death between buns. Don't eat them. Instead, make your own with lean ground beef, buffalo, or turkey.

For the best ground beef burger, buy a lean cut of sirloin or round and have the butcher grind it for you. You can also read the labels of the packaged ground beef and get the one with the lowest fat content.

TAKE THIS THOUGHT TO BED WITH YOU

Everything that is worthwhile is worth waiting for. Relax and take several deep breaths. Think about how good it feels to just sink back and relax. Let your body's energy flow freely through you. Think of times that made you particularly happy, and hold on to those thoughts as you drift off to sleep.

Do it! Write it! Be it!

WHAT YOU ATE (If you swallowed it, write it down)

Breakfast: Lunch: Supper:

_____   _____   _____

_____   _____   _____

_____   _____   _____

_____   _____   _____

_____   _____   _____

_____   _____   _____

_____   _____   _____

Snacks:

WHAT YOU DID

Cardiovascular Exercise	Time	Notes
_____	_____	_____
_____	_____	_____
_____	_____	_____

Side Twists	Reps/Sets	Notes
_____	_____	_____
_____	_____	_____

Other Activities

_____

_____

_____

_____

_____

WHAT YOU THOUGHT

ONLY 8 DAYS TO GO!

DAY 21

BRAIN POWER

Think of your alarm clock as an opportunity clock! Then open the curtains and pull up the shades on a brand new day and a brand new you!

The finish line is in sight. Did you know you'd make it this far? Do you like the changes the program has brought? Are you getting compliments from people around you about the bounce in your step, the color in your cheeks, and that starting-to-slim-down new look?

Be selfish! Reap all the rewards you can! Accept all the applause, because today it's show time!

Whether it's for church or a lunch with friends or relatives, dress up today and show off the new you. You've put so much into yourself these last three weeks that now it's time to try on some new clothes and step out your door looking, and feeling, your absolute best!

EATING RIGHT

Take small bites. Eat slowly and savor your food. Drink plenty of water with meals. You'll feel full faster. Remember, water, water, water!

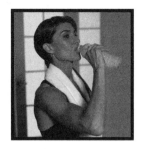

BREAKFAST

Breakfast on the go: You know what to reach for: a high-protein, low-carbohydrate meal replacement smoothie, shake, or bar. Add a piece of fruit and water. Remember to obey your thirst!

Sit-down breakfast: Take your pick of two or three eggs or a nice slice of lean meat, ground turkey burger, or soy burger. Add a side of cottage cheese and two pieces of rye toast with all-fruit spread or almond butter. Finish it off with sliced apples, pears, or apricots. Be sure to drink at least one glass of water, nonfat milk, or tea or coffee with your meal.

LUNCH

Lunch on the go: Have an open-faced deli sandwich with chicken or turkey and cheese, no mayonnaise, and a three-bean or pasta salad on the side. Drink plenty of water.

Sit-down lunch: Make a couple of bean burritos with extra lettuce or concoct a generous chunky chicken salad, fajita salad, or Cobb salad without the bacon. Use lots of greens. Use no more than two tablespoons of dressing. Finish off with a piece of fruit and a large glass of water or iced tea.

SUPPER

Supper on the go: Grab a fist-sized portion of lean meat from the deli and enjoy with a cup of lentil or split pea soup, or a three-bean or pasta salad. Enjoy a low-fat, low-sugar yogurt, preferably plain, with nuts or fresh fruit for dessert, and water.

Sit-down supper: Indulge yourself with a generous fist-sized lean meat or protein source, plus fist-sized portions of vegetables and low-glycemic carbohydrates. Finish with a low-fat, low-sugar yogurt, preferably plain, mixed with nuts and your favorite fruit. Don't forget to drink plenty of water.

Or, go out to eat and have somebody else fix supper for you, the way you want it. Have a single glass of red wine, if you like, with a healthy meal and no dishes to clean.

WORKOUT

No formal exercise today. Relax. You've taken care of yourself all week. Maybe you should find some things to do around the house. Sunday chores always seem to be waiting for you—clean out a closet, the garage, or your car. Remember, these aren't formal exercises but they are calorie burners just the same so keep track of them, and your thoughts about the last two weeks of touch workouts.

We're social animals. Call a friend or relative you haven't spoken to in a long time. Tell them about our one-on-one program and the results you've been achieving. Take pride in your accomplishments.

Good health is contagious. Spread it around!

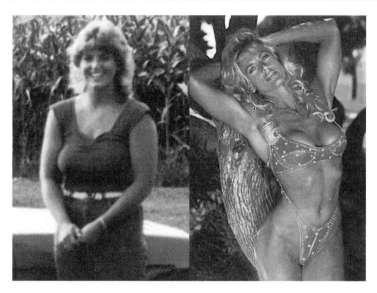

*Tony's knowledge and guidance helped
Jana Garry from Indiana lose 60 stubborn pounds
and get into the best shape of her life.
She's now a fitness model!*

HEALTH SMARTS

STRESS CAN MAKE YOU FAT, OR, *IF YOU WORRY, YOU DIE EARLY*

Stress produces chemical changes that may lead to weight gain—particularly around the waist—and prevent you from being the best you can be.

Stress comes in many forms: financial worries, family problems, too much or too little work, love lost, a new love, marriage, a new baby, new jobs and accidents, just to name a few. When you are under stress as a result of either internal or external pressures, your body secretes stress hormones known as "catecholamines." These chemicals prepare the body for what is called the "fight-or-flight" response.

Recent research has shown that women may respond differently to this traditional emergency response with a "tend and nurture" response, but the chemical effects are still the same. Whether we tend, fight, nurture, or flee, the same chemicals are activated within our bodies.

When you are under stress, a cascade of catecholamines is produced. Your muscles become tense, your heart rate increases, and your blood pressure rises. Your blood sugar levels spike upward, providing you with a quick source of energy. The stomach and intestines slow down their activities. These physical changes are accompanied by psychological responses such as anxiety, inability to focus your thoughts, inability to sleep, and perhaps even a sense of panic.

A noted study linking stress to immune dysfunction was done in 1991, when Carnegie Mellon psychologist Sheldon Cohen and his colleagues showed that people who ranked high on a psychological test of perceived stress were more likely to develop colds when intentionally infected with a respiratory virus.

In 1998, Cohen repeated the study and this time refined his results. Although a single, large, stressful event in the preceding year did not affect the subjects' chances of getting sick, chronic stress—ongoing conflicts with coworkers or family members, for example—increased the odds by as much as three to five times.

Stress Can Kill

In addition to causing colds and flu, stress and anxiety contribute to a wide variety of other conditions and diseases, some even fatal, such as heart disease and cancer, according to the National Institutes of Health (NIH) and other major research centers.

Chronic stress influences the cardiovascular, immune, and nervous systems. Chronic stress can damage the heart in a number of ways. Something as simple as doing intense mental calculations or being in a physically uncomfortable situation can increase blood pressure. Extreme stress can lead to heart palpitations, fibrillation, and even death.

Stress Can Also Make You Fat

Chronic stress produces a constant flood of the stress hormone cortisol. Abnormally prolonged cortisol secretion stimulates the hormone insulin. During chronic stress, insulin, a powerful fat storage hormone, short-circuits the release of fat and encourages fat storage, especially inside the abdomen.

Young and middle-aged adults who gain excess weight are at highest risk for insulin resistance and a condition known as hyperinsulinemia. One study concluded that each 5% increase in weight gain over age 20 was accompanied by an almost 20% greater incidence of insulin resistance. Even without dramatic weight gain, an age-associated trend toward hyperinsulinemia and insulin resistance has been identified. In fact, research reveals that from 10% to 25% of the U.S. population may be insulin resistant. With recent statistics stating that 61% of the United States is overweight and 29% is obese, there could actually be even more Americans who are insulin resistant.

Therefore, since under stress you are burning less fat, chronic stress can literally make you fat, especially around your stomach!

Exercise: A Powerful Antidote to Stress

In addition to taking over-the-counter herbal remedies or prescription drugs to control anxiety, doing cardioexercise is essential for stress reduction. In a *Newsweek* cover story on stress, researchers found that after a half-hour on a treadmill, exercisers scored 25% lower on anxiety tests and exhibited favorable changes in brain activity. "Physical activity bathes the body with soothing brain chemicals, which is nature's way of saying 'Relax. The predator is gone,' " notes University of Maryland stress physiology expert Pamela Peeke, MD, MPH, in her book *Fight Fat After 40*.

Even people who stress out easily can learn to moderate their responses. At the University of Massachusetts Center for Mindfulness in Medicine, Health Care and Society, specialists have spent some 20 years teaching people to manage stress through meditation, yoga, and other relaxation exercises.

During their weekly sessions, participants in the center's stress program concentrate on breathing to quell the mind's obsession with the past and future. Then they lie down and mentally scan their bodies, relaxing one muscle at a time. Studies suggest that this type of exercise can reduce the flow of stress hormones, helping to lower both heart rate and blood pressure. Massage is another proven way of reducing stress.

Other options such as Tai Chi, biofeedback, music therapy, or all of these combined, reduce stress significantly. So does writing in a journal or seeking help in a support group. The key, experts agree, is that all of these activities combat feelings of helplessness and stop you from feeling like a victim.

Because no single activity or remedy can keep your stress at bay, it's important to engage in a combination of solutions. These include herbal and prescription remedies, regular exercise, meditation, massages, journal writing, and talking to friends. All of these can help you conquer stress and live a healthier, happier life.

TAKE THIS THOUGHT TO BED WITH YOU

Three weeks into the program and you're practically a walking encyclopedia on good health habits!

Why not share some of that knowledge with a friend? Ask them over to your house for a workout one morning or for an outdoor walk. Show them the book and your progress logs. If you belong to a health club, invite your friend along for a trial workout.

For good health to truly become a lifestyle, you'll need to meet other people who share your interest and can continue to exchange information on how they stay on track and stay feeling fit and young.

Surround yourself with healthy books and magazines as well; the book you're reading now is a terrific place to begin your collection. Read the newspaper for interesting pieces on health and new research, and stay abreast of the news that's out there. Stay away from negative people, hang out with positive people.

The better informed you are, the better off you'll be *for life!*

Do it! Write it! Be it!

WHAT YOU ATE (If you swallowed it, write it down)

Breakfast: Lunch: Supper:

_____   _____   _____
_____   _____   _____
_____   _____   _____
_____   _____   _____
_____   _____   _____
_____   _____   _____
_____   _____   _____

Snacks:

WHAT YOU DID

Cardiovascular Exercise   Time   Notes

_____   _____   _____
_____   _____   _____
_____   _____   _____
_____   _____   _____

Other Exercise

_____
_____
_____
_____
_____
_____
_____

WHAT YOU THOUGHT

_____
_____
_____
_____
_____
_____
_____
_____
_____
_____
_____
_____
_____
_____
_____
_____
_____
_____
_____
_____
_____
_____
_____
_____
_____
_____
_____
_____

ONLY 7 DAYS TO GO!

WEEK 4:
The Home Stretch

5

> If you've followed the program to this point, today you are a different person than three weeks ago. You've empowered yourself with accomplishment. Now if you continue to reaffirm the positive changes you've experienced, you will continue to benefit. Look in your logs. You did it. It worked. Keep doing it.

DAY 22

BRAIN POWER

Take a lesson from babies and animals. Most wake up happy. Babies smile, kittens cuddle, and birds sing in the trees. Remember that when you wake up: be happy. Laugh often. Laugh long. Laugh loud. Laugh until you have to gasp for breath. Do that every day, and you will be a better person for it.

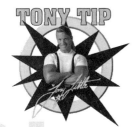

Look back through your logs and make a list of all the good things you've learned, done, and felt in the past 21 days. Take as much time as you need to make this list. Check how your body has changed, how your clothes fit. Then put the list up on your bathroom mirror and add to it as your final week comes to a close.

When you began this program you knew what you wanted; you just didn't know how to get it. Now you do. Believe in the program. Believe in yourself. You will succeed.

EATING RIGHT

This is probably becoming second nature to you now, but here are some suggestions for this final week.

BREAKFAST

Breakfast on the go: If you are a person on the go or someone who doesn't usually eat breakfast, reach for a high-protein, low-carbohydrate meal replacement smoothie or bar. Remember to drink at least eight ounces of water with breakfast, and don't forget a multiple vitamin/mineral supplement.

Sit-down breakfast: Poach, fry with Pam spray, or scramble three eggs (or egg substitute). Enjoy this with two slices of sourdough or rye bread with I Can't Believe It's Not Butter spray or a trans-fat-free spread. Drink one cup of coffee or tea, no sugar, black or with a low-fat cream substitute. You may also have a six-ounce glass of orange juice or apple juice or a piece of fruit.

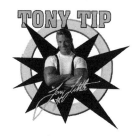

LUNCH

Lunch on the go: Head off to Subway for a variety of healthy low-fat sandwiches and salads. Or, go to the deli and select lean meat, with light or no mayonnaise, and rye or whole-grain bread.

Sit-down lunch: Fix yourself a Boca burger. These veggie burgers are the best. Prepare with light mayonnaise (if you must) and ketchup, lettuce, tomato, and onion and put it all between two slices of whole-grain bread. A little steak sauce makes it like a barbecued delight! Add a slice of low-fat cheese or a couple slices of avocado, and you've got a great lunch.

Have dried, canned, or fresh apricots for dessert. Drink at least eight ounces of water.

SUPPER

Supper on the go: Hold the mayonnaise on a deli sandwich of either chicken or turkey and wash it down with a berry smoothie.

Sit-down supper: A fist-sized portion of chicken, fish, lean beef, or soy with a fist-sized portion of beans, pasta, noodles, or rice. Add a fist-sized portion of green peas, corn, green beans, raw carrots, or spinach. Enjoy trail mix with nuts and dried fruit for dessert, but don't get the type with carob and yogurt chips. Drink lots of water!

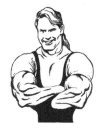 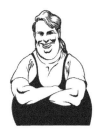

Tony walks the walk and it shows.
If he just talked the talk, it would show too!
Illustration by Matt Gouig

> **Y**ou can't just give lip service to your workout and nutritional plans. You've got to put them in action. Make them a habit. You're already well on your way!

WORKOUT

Here's the drill for the rest of the program: six days cardio, three days resistance, plus three extra ab days. Let's get movin'.

CARDIOVASCULAR EXERCISE

Let's really push ourselves. For those of you who feel up to it, strive for 30 to 45 minutes of cardio this week. As I said before, we have weak and strong days. When you feel that you can go to 45 minutes, go for it! The more you put in, the more you get back. It's for you!

Let's do some more interval cardio. Begin with marching in place (lift those knees high), then follow with some easy stretches. As you start your cardio, watch the clock and speed your pace up a notch at 15-second intervals, until you are breathing hard. Remember: keep your movements fluid, energized, and brisk—not fast, just comfortable. If you feel you're breathing too hard, check your Target Heart Rate (see Day 9). After this, proceed with your favorite cardio activity for the duration of the time you've chosen. Don't forget the Two-Minute Warning, then really crank up the pace faster and harder than ever before. Cool down for five minutes with light marching in place.

> **T**he benefits of cardio conditioning begin showing up immediately. Look how far you've come so far! The benefits also stay with you an average of two months, so as you progress, you can cut back on your cardio days without losing the conditioning. However, cardio does burn a lot of calories and you should keep it up until you've reached your weight goal.

RESISTANCE EXERCISE

Here we go again. A different arrangement of the exercises you've already learned, plus some new ones to tone you up and lean you out!

DAY 22

For this workout, which you can do at home, you will need some light dumbbells in whatever weights you feel comfortable with. If you do not have weights, try soup cans! But by now, I hope you have some weights!

1. Full squat (front and back of upper legs and butt):

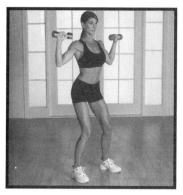 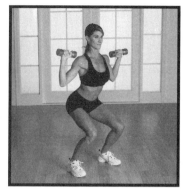

For at home or at the gym. Stand with your feet shoulder-width apart, dumbbells held at shoulder height. Now slowly lower yourself as if you were about to sit in a chair. Go as far down as you're comfortable, ideally until your thighs are parallel to the floor. Use the same weight or a little heavier than last week.

> **SET ONE:** 10–15 repetitions
> **SET TWO:** 10–15 repetitions
> **SET THREE:** 10–15 repetitions

1a. Leg press machine (front of upper legs and butt):

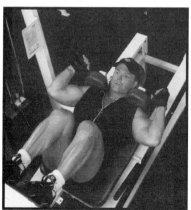 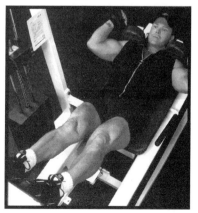

For the gym only. Position the machine so that your knees are bent and you're a little squished at the start. The first portion of this exercise hits the glutes and creates a great looking butt! Push your legs out until they are straight, but don't lock the knees. Then return, under control, to the starting position. Use the same weight as last week.

SET ONE: 10–15 repetitions
SET TWO: 10–15 repetitions
SET THREE: 10–15 repetitions

2. Stationary lunge (hamstrings, gluteals)

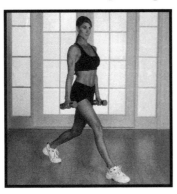 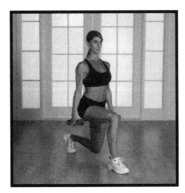

For at home or at the gym. Use light dumbbells in your hands for this. Perform by standing upright and taking a large stride forward with your right leg. This is the start position. Let your left knee trail as low as comfortable, but do not touch the floor. Keep your forward knee over the ball of your foot. If it extends too far, your stride is too short. If it doesn't go over the ball of your foot, your stride is too long. Stand back up to the start position. Think *squeeze*. Finish all your reps for one leg before moving to the other leg.

SET ONE: 8–10 repetitions
SET TWO: 8–10 repetitions
SET THREE: 8–10 repetitions

2a. Leg extension (front of upper legs):

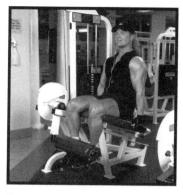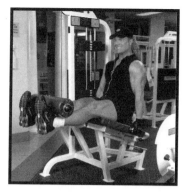

For the gym only. Position yourself in a leg extension machine so the front of your ankles are secure behind the pads. Hold onto the side handles. Squeeze your quads as you extend your legs straight out in front of you. Hold for one second at the peak contraction, then lower the bar. Try to increase your weight from last week on at least one set.

> **SET ONE:** 10–15 repetitions
> **SET TWO:** 10–15 repetitions
> **SET THREE:** 10–15 repetitions

3. Wide-stance squat (legs, inner thighs):

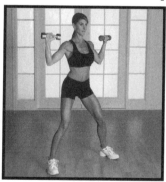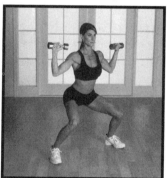

For at home or at the gym. Holding two dumbbells at shoulder height, stand with your feet wider apart than shoulder width, toes pointed out at ten and two o'clock. Keep your back straight and eyes up, then squat down as far as comfortable. Then push back up with your legs. Perform this slowly, using a four-count on the way down and a three-count on the way up. *Squeeze* your glutes!

> **SET ONE:** 10–15 repetitions
> **SET TWO:** 10–15 repetitions
> **SET THREE:** 10–15 repetitions

3a. Leg press machine (quads, hamstrings, inner thighs):

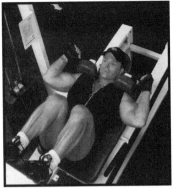
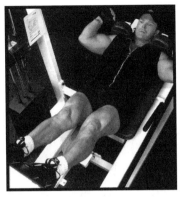

For the gym only. This versatile machine lets you focus on different parts of your upper leg musculature. To imitate the inner thigh work on the wide-stance squat, just place your feet out to the corners of the pads. If your feet are closer together, it better imitates the full squat. Begin by pushing the platform up past the slide guards. Be certain the weight is under your control at all times. With abs, arms, and legs tense, lower the weight as far as comfortable and without reversing the motion and push back to the top while squeezing your muscles.

> **SET ONE:** 10–15 repetitions
> **SET TWO:** 10–15 repetitions
> **SET THREE:** 10–15 repetitions

4. Back Row with chair (v-taper of back):

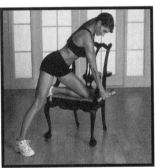
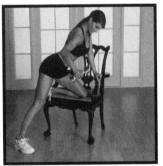
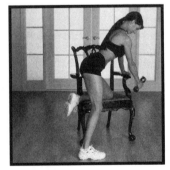

For at home or at the gym. This is a great exercise for strengthening the back. At home, find a sturdy armless chair and kneel on it as shown. In the gym, use a bench. Try and keep your chest almost parallel to the floor and your back straight, balance on the chair with one arm and hold a dumbbell (use a light, 5- to 20-pound dumbbell) at arm's length in the other hand. Keeping your upper body tense, squeeze the dumbbell up to the side of your chest, elbow slightly bent out, then return to arm's length and stretch (but not to the floor).

SET ONE: 10–15 repetitions
SET TWO: 10–15 repetitions
SET THREE: 10–15 repetitions

4a. Back row machine (back):

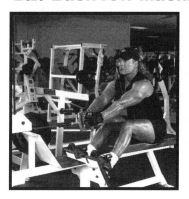 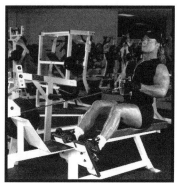

For the gym only. Grab the close-grip handles on a rowing machine with a 45-degree back, then push back with your legs until there is tension on the cable. From this position, pull the handles close to your body and squeeze your shoulder blades at the peak of the movement. Return to the original position.

SET ONE: 10–15 repetitions
SET TWO: 10–15 repetitions
SET THREE: 10–15 repetitions

5. Chest crossover (chest):

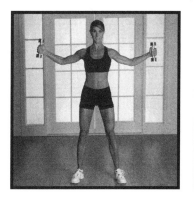 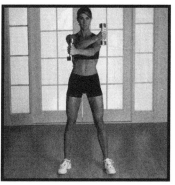

For at home or at the gym. Hold a dumbbell in each hand, arms outstretched to your sides. As though you were hugging a barrel, bring the dumbbells together in front of you, *squeeze,* top arm over. For the next rep, switch to other arm over.

DAY 22

SET ONE: 10–15 repetitions
SET TWO: 10–15 repetitions
SET THREE: 10–15 repetitions

5a. Chest machine or pec deck (chest):

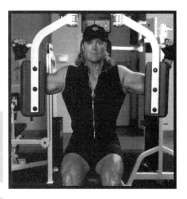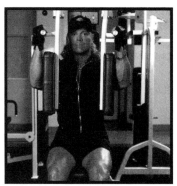

For the gym only. Position the seat so that your forearms are firmly against the pads. With a light grip on the handles squeeze down on your chest muscles and bring the handles together in front of you. Hold for a moment (squeezing) and return to the start. This exercise works the inside of the chest, or the cleavage. Caution: never extend your elbows behind your shoulders.

SET ONE: 10–15 repetitions
SET TWO: 10–15 repetitions
SET THREE: 10–15 repetitions

HEALTH SMARTS

THE POWER OF BELIEF

No need to light the candles or rattle the beads. This is no hocus-pocus. It's just the gosh-darn truth.

The mind and the body work together. Positive thinking and belief in your ability not only can get you in shape and keep you in shape but also can actually heal you.

Mental stress, fatigue, and grief can lead to illness and disease. Mental energy makes your workouts more productive. And these are proven medical facts.

The power of the mind in healing has been recognized since the dawn of man. Let us not overlook the tales of Jesus returning sight and the use of a limb, or those fabled medicine women, ancient shamans, and other religious leaders who have long been credited with healing powers that involved no drugs or surgery.

People who deal with illness and pain know full well that a patient may feel relief simply by being in their caregivers' presence, if they are positive and assuring. Long before placebos had a name, healers would apply soothing salves and offer warm broth to bring comfort to a patient. When a patient truly believed these herbs were medicinal in nature, the relief often led to healing.

Scientifically Proven

Recent studies have consistently found that 30% to 40% of all patients given a placebo show improvement for a wide variety of symptoms and conditions. These include coughing, nausea, dental pain, angina, migraine, and even ulcers. Even more interesting is the fact that about 10% of people given a placebo report side effects normally associated with a chemically active drug.

Placebos work best when certain conditions are met. First, the patients must believe that someone is truly trying to help them. They must expect to find relief in the therapy. If the caregiver is extremely optimistic and works in a clinical setting, the placebo effect of a sugar pill is enhanced.

Heal Thyself

There is strong scientific support that the mind and body work together and the power of belief can heal. This evidence does not mean that drugs, surgery, and other treatments don't work. It also does not imply that belief is all that is required to heal. But faith can work miracles.

This program is not a placebo! It will work, even if you only go through the motions!

But if you believe in this program, it will not only work but *it will work wonders*.

It is important that you believe, so that you continue, day by day, to make this program work. Without faith, men and women are not much different than wild beasts.

Believe. Imagine. You will achieve.

TAKE THIS THOUGHT TO BED WITH YOU

Alrighty! You are officially a weight trainer now. If you have been doing this program in the gym, look around and remember how awkward the first days were, and how comfortable you feel now. That's because you're with your peers! If you trained at home, I bet you feel a little bit better off than your friends who haven't gotten bitten by the fitness bug. Share the book. Share your success. It will fuel even bigger and better things.

Don't forget to stretch!

You worked hard. Sleep well.

Do it! Write it! Be it!

WHAT YOU ATE (If you swallowed it, write it down)

Breakfast: Lunch: Supper:

_____   _____   _____
_____   _____   _____
_____   _____   _____
_____   _____   _____
_____   _____   _____
_____   _____   _____
_____   _____   _____
_____   _____   _____

Snacks:

WHAT YOU DID

Cardiovascular Exercise   Time   Notes

_____   _____   _____
_____   _____   _____

Resistance Exercise   Reps/Sets/Weight   Notes

_____   _____   _____
_____   _____   _____
_____   _____   _____
_____   _____   _____
_____   _____   _____
_____   _____   _____
_____   _____   _____
_____   _____   _____

WHAT YOU THOUGHT

_____
_____
_____
_____
_____
_____
_____
_____
_____
_____
_____
_____
_____
_____
_____
_____
_____
_____
_____
_____
_____
_____
_____
_____

ONLY 6 DAYS TO GO!

DAY 23

Always live for today. There really is no beginning or end. Yesterday is history and tomorrow is a mystery. Today is a gift that should be opened and enjoyed all day long.

EATING RIGHT

Have you stocked up on some of those Boca burgers? They make a quick snack on their own, with a little steak sauce or ketchup and low-fat cottage cheese and a piece of fruit on the side. Keep them on hand.

BREAKFAST

Breakfast on the go: Reach for a balanced meal replacement. For in-between hunger attacks, how about a fist-sized portion of lean deli meat or a hard-boiled egg?

Sit-down breakfast: Time for another south-of-the-border burrito for the extra thermogenic properties that help burn calories! Use a reduced-fat tortilla and add sautéed fresh vegetables, two or three eggs or tofu, salsa, and hot peppers to taste. Enjoy with one slice of whole-grain, rye or pumpernickel bread and a cup of coffee or tea.

LUNCH

Lunch on the go: A meal replacement with fresh fruit, carrots, and plenty of water! Or, a quick trip to Taco Bell for plain bean burritos or soft chicken tacos.

Sit-down lunch: Make a sandwich with two slices of sourdough or rye bread, a fist-sized portion of lean meat or a grilled portobello mushroom, a dab of low-fat mayonnaise, a slice of avocado, some lettuce or sprouts and a slice of tomato.

Have an apple or two apricots for dessert. Drink at least eight ounces of water.

SUPPER

Supper on the go: Heat up a low-sodium soup—lentil, green pea, bean, or barley—or a low-carb, high-protein smoothie or meal replacement bar, and enjoy with one or two slices of rye or pumpernickel bread and lots of water!

Sit-down supper: Choose a fist-sized portion of lean meat or a soy burger, grilled. Now go to my list of low-glycemic carbohydrates and choose two fist-sized portions of vegetables (yellow, green, or red) and another carbohydrate, plus one piece of fruit.

Always drink plenty of water with your meals.

WORKOUT

Today it's 30 to 45 minutes of cardio and a couple of ab moves. Pick your favorite cardio, crank up the music, and get your body moving! You're in your fat-burning mode!

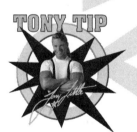

Your improved conditioning level is helping your body to more efficiently burn calories and build lean muscle. Keep the momentum going and changes will begin to come much faster.

CARDIOVASCULAR EXERCISE

The same 30 to 45 minutes, but do it at an interval pace. Speed it up for a minute or two every five to six minutes, then cool back down. Interval is the most effective kind of cardio for burning calories. Also, energize your mind and emotions with some loud music you love!

RESISTANCE EXERCISE

Today involves stretching and some more work for your abs.

1. Ab crunch (upper abdominals):

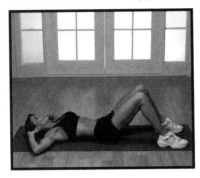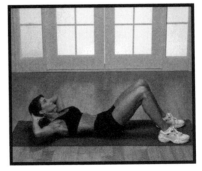

For at home or at the gym. Keep your body as tense as possible and keep these movements slow and precise. Think *squeeze* and technique! For variety, perform these on a large exercise ball.

SET ONE: 10–20 repetitions
SET TWO: 10–20 repetitions
SET THREE: 10–20 repetitions

2. Compound crunch (abdominals):

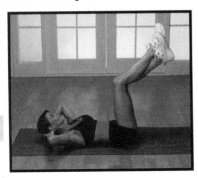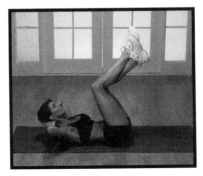

For at home or at the gym. This move works both the upper and lower portions of the abs. Perform these until failure (the point at which you just can't do any more). Push yourself for more!

SET ONE: 10–20 repetitions
SET TWO: 10–20 repetitions
SET THREE: 10–20 repetitions

3. Reverse crunch (abdominals):

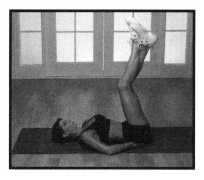 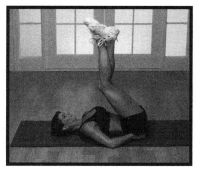

For at home or at the gym. Lie on your back with your hands under the small of your back. Keeping your back pressed to your hands, rock your hips up and tuck your knees in to your shoulders. Your hips should come up from the mat, but not your lower back.

> **SET ONE:** 10–20 repetitions
> **SET TWO:** 10–20 repetitions
> **SET THREE:** 10–20 repetitions

HEALTH SMARTS

AVERTING AND LIVING WITH BACK PAIN

My three serious car accidents have left my lower back a mess. But these experiences have also made me quite an expert on dealing with problematic backs. In any case, you don't have to be in three major wrecks to wreck your back. Back pain affects more than 80% of Americans. It seems that if you live long enough, your turn will come.

The reasons for the pain are varied. Poor posture, poor lifting technique, or a degenerative disk disease can all lead to lower back pain.

The best way to avoid back pain is to never strain your back. That also means never playing golf, never playing tennis, or never doing other sports and being a weenie by never lifting anything heavier than ten pounds. Even if you practice proper lifting techniques, there will be situations where you need to move an object that's out in front of your body. Just tucking in a baby at night puts a bad strain on your back.

Back extensions, which I recommend throughout my program, are good strengtheners to protect the lower back. The hip circles I suggested from Chinese medicine can also help. Correcting your posture, standing taller, and not allowing yourself to "rest" on your spine is also a big plus in eliminating back pain. If you run, never do so on pavement, and choose grass or track instead. If you have back pain, avoid running uphill.

Anyone with back pain should avoid standing while taking their shoes off. Sit down and make certain your back is stable. Even if you don't have back pain, sitting to put your shoes on is a good idea.

My workouts include several movements to improve back strength. Strong muscles can help protect disks from injury. Never exercise your back if it hurts; exercise it when it feels healthy and stop as soon as pain shows itself.

If you're a woman, stop wearing high heels, right now! They distort your posture so that too much strain is put on your lower back.

If you injure your back, massage is good and I do believe in chiropractors as long as they are gentle. Use the R.I.C.E. method to relieve pain—that is, Rest, Ice, Compression, and Elevate. Immediately apply ice and rest. Do not continue once your back is sore. Do not apply heat in the first 24 hours, and then moist heat after that. Sports medicine clinics are also good sources of rehabilitative care. Surgery should always be your last resort.

The best thing you can do for yourself is what you are already doing: following a weekly plan of balanced exercise. Lift smart in your workouts, and lift smart in your home.

TAKE THIS THOUGHT TO BED WITH YOU

You are working like a true athlete right now. Look back through your logs and see how your thinking has progressed. Are you expecting more from yourself? Okay, you're doing it. I knew you could!

Sleep deep. Dream big.

Do it! Write it! Be it!

WHAT YOU ATE (If you swallowed it, write it down)

Breakfast: Lunch: Supper:

_____   _____   _____
_____   _____   _____
_____   _____   _____
_____   _____   _____
_____   _____   _____
_____   _____   _____
_____   _____   _____

Snacks:

WHAT YOU DID

Cardiovascular Exercise   Time   Notes

_____   _____   _____
_____   _____   _____
_____   _____   _____

Resistance Exercise   Reps/Sets   Notes

_____   _____   _____
_____   _____   _____
_____   _____   _____

Other Exercise

_____
_____
_____
_____

WHAT YOU THOUGHT

ONLY 5 DAYS TO GO!

DAY 24

BRAIN POWER

Heroes and heroines have blazed their way through history. Many stood alone against great odds. Many sacrificed their lives for strangers and ignored danger to save others. The world is built upon the courage of millions of forgotten people whose bravery has given life and hope to others. Before your life is done, be that kind of hero. It's as simple as touching one other person with the gift of good health.

EATING RIGHT

You know this drill by now. Take my suggestions or fill in on your own.

BREAKFAST

Breakfast on the go: Reach for your usual staple of meal replacements, or eat low-fat, low-sugar yogurt, preferably plain, and a piece of fruit with your coffee, tea, or water.

Sit-down breakfast: Scramble two or three eggs with American or cheddar cheese. Have three slices of turkey bacon or lean ham and two slices of rye, sourdough, or pumpernickel bread. Drink a glass of apple juice, or coffee or tea, no sugar, black or with a low-fat cream substitute. Are you full and happy? Now get yourself off to a really productive day. Make every second count!

LUNCH

Lunch on the go: How about some Chinese takeout today? Ask for no or low oil and no MSG. Stay away from batter-dipped meals and the sweet and sour. Good choices include spring vegetables with bean curd, broccoli and chicken, and black bean chicken. Order steamed rice instead of fried.

Sit-down lunch: Make a sandwich of sourdough, rye, or pumpernickel bread with light mayonnaise, a dab of mustard, and your choice of lean deli meat. Add lettuce, cheese, and tomato for a high-protein, low-carbohydrate lunch. Have an apple or orange for dessert.

Drink at least eight ounces of water.

SUPPER

Supper on the go: Grab a big meal replacement shake or smoothie with an extra scoop of protein powder. Enjoy with two pieces of fresh fruit, half a cantaloupe, or apple or pear slices.

Sit-down supper: Grill or broil a fist-sized portion of cube steak (you may substitute tuna steak, salmon, chicken breast, or turkey), and add a fist-sized portion of green beans, lima beans, spinach, or salad with oil and vinegar, fat-free Italian dressing, or balsamic vinegar. Have one sweet or baked potato with light butter or trans-fat-free spread (read the label). Try a bit of A-1 sauce on your potato.

Again, drink plenty of water.

WORKOUT

Here we go again with cardio and calorie-burning, big muscle-resistance training. Gear up, it's a big day!

CARDIOVASCULAR EXERCISE

Go for 30 to 45 minutes of your favorite cardio today. Remember our Perceived Rate of Exertion (PRE)? Well on a scale of 1 to 10, that should be around 6 to 8 now. Think about some interval spurts to keep it going!

RESISTANCE EXERCISE

Jump in and go for it!

This is the last week. Challenge yourself, but don't forget your *squeeze* technique!

1. Wide-stance squat (legs, inner thighs):

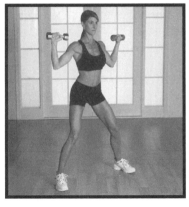
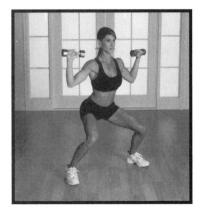

For at home or at the gym. Stand with your feet wider apart than shoulder width, toes pointed out at ten and two o'clock. Keep your back straight and eyes up and squat down as far as comfortable. *Squeeze* your glutes!

> **SET ONE:** 10–15 repetitions
> **SET TWO:** 10–15 repetitions
> **SET THREE:** 10–15 repetitions

1a. Leg press machine (quads, hamstrings, inner thighs):

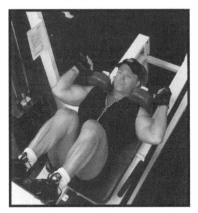
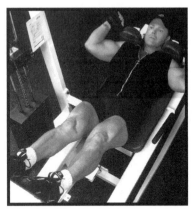

For the gym only. Begin by pushing the platform up past the slide guards. Once you remove these guards, the machine has the capability to come nearly all the way down. Be certain the weight is under your control. With abs, arms, and legs tense, lower the weight as far as comfortable and without reversing the motion.

> **SET ONE:** 10–15 repetitions
> **SET TWO:** 10–15 repetitions
> **SET THREE:** 10–15 repetitions

DAY 24

2. Walking lunge (back of upper legs and butt):

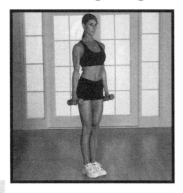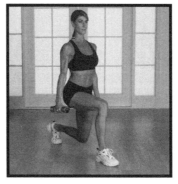

For at home or at the gym. Stand upright and take a large stride forward with your right leg. Let your left knee trail as low as comfortable, but do not touch the floor. Now begin to stand upright and take another stride with your left leg—as if you are walking. Count each step as one rep and strive for the recommended reps or until failure.

SET ONE: 20–25 repetitions
SET TWO: 20–25 repetitions

2a. Leg extension (quadriceps):

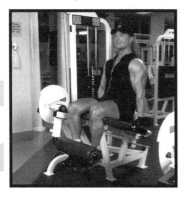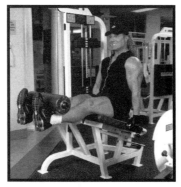

For the gym only. Position yourself in a leg extension machine so the front of your ankles are secure behind the pads. Hold onto the side handles. Squeeze your quads as you extend your legs straight out in front of you. Hold for one second at the peak contraction, *squeeze,* then lower the bar.

SET ONE: 10–15 repetitions
SET TWO: 10–15 repetitions
SET THREE: 10–15 repetitions

3. Back Row with chair (v-taper of back):

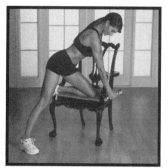 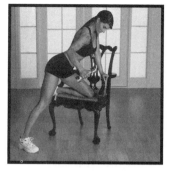 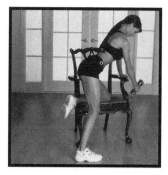

For at home or at the gym. This is a great exercise for strengthening the back. At home, find a sturdy armless chair and kneel on it as shown. In the gym, use a bench. Try and keep your chest almost parallel to the floor and your back straight, balance on the chair with one arm and hold a dumbbell (use a light, 5- to 20-pound dumbbell) at arm's length in the other hand. Keeping your upper body tense, squeeze the dumbbell up to the side of your chest, elbow slightly bent out, then return to arm's length and stretch (but not to the floor).

> **SET ONE:** 10–15 repetitions
> **SET TWO:** 10–15 repetitions
> **SET THREE:** 10–15 repetitions

3a. Lat pulldown (back):

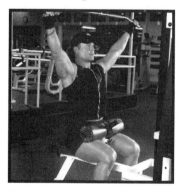 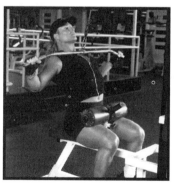

For the gym only. Any wide grip used in a pulling motion exercises the large muscles that run along the sides of the back. Position yourself so your knees are secure under the pads. Reach up and take a wide grip on the bar. Squeeze your back muscles as you pull the bar down to your upper chest, arching slightly. Return completely under your control.

DAY 24

SET ONE: 10–15 repetitions
SET TWO: 10–15 repetitions
SET THREE: 10–15 repetitions

4. Modified push-up or push-up (chest):

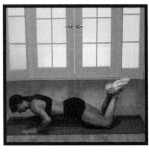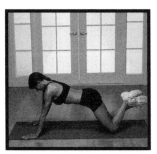
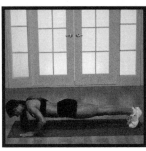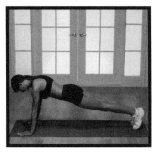

For at home or at the gym. You may perform this according to your conditioning. The easiest way is to perform it leaning against a table-high object. A more difficult push-up may be done lying flat on the floor and pushing up from your knees (as shown). The hardest form of push-up is lying flat on your stomach and pushing your entire body up from the floor while only your hands and toes are touching the floor. In all the different variations, your hands should be positioned just outside your shoulders, arms slightly bent out, elbows in line with your shoulders, back straight, and your neck in a neutral position. Lower down to the point just before your chest touches the floor and then squeeze your chest muscles as you raise up, repeat.

SET ONE: 10–15 repetitions
SET TWO: 10–15 repetitions
SET THREE: 10–15 repetitions

4a. Chest press machine (chest):

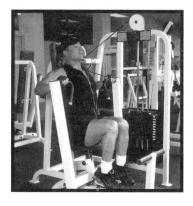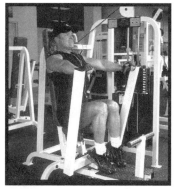

For the gym only. With your feet firmly on the pad, tense your upper body, particularly your chest, and push the weight directly in front of you. Hold for one-half second at the peak contraction, then return under control.

SET ONE: 10–15 repetitions
SET TWO: 10–15 repetitions
SET THREE: 10–15 repetitions

HEALTH SMARTS

DIET AND HEART DISEASE

There is no question that the American diet is to blame for our country's high incidence of heart disease. Many of the same diet factors that contribute to heart disease also contribute to excess weight gain. No wonder the average American is hit with the double whammy of being overweight and at risk of heart disease!

Lowering saturated fat will go a long way in helping you lower your total fat and total calories in order to lose weight. As an added benefit, lowering your saturated fat will also help reduce your risk of heart disease.

If you have a family history of heart disease, if you smoke, if you are overweight and overstressed, you should definitely have your cholesterol checked by a physician to determine if you need to make even more drastic changes to your diet. Even if you don't suffer from any of the above, it's always a good idea to have a cholesterol test.

Fat Versus Cholesterol

Cholesterol is a thick, waxy fat that is often confused with dietary fat. Advertisers often contribute to the confusion to try and sell their products. Here's an example.

Shrimp is full of cholesterol, but it's okay, even healthy, to eat shrimp. A slyly packaged "cholesterol-free" cookie, however, has fat and may contribute greatly to a buildup of artery-clogging fat that can eventually choke off the supply of blood to the heart.

Much of the confusion comes from the fact that consumption of saturated fats, not consumption of cholesterol, is what contributes to the buildup of cholesterol in the arteries and leads to heart disease. Food manufacturers know this fact, so they label many foods "cholesterol-free," even though the foods contain saturated fats that when consumed, raise the level of heart disease–causing cholesterol in your blood.

Saturated fat and cholesterol are high in most red meats, liver, organ meats, and dairy products, including whole milk, butter, eggs, and cheese. Coconut and palm oil are nearly 100% saturated fat. Saturated fat is usually solid at refrigerator temperature. It needs to be eaten in moderation.

On the other hand, monounsaturated and polyunsaturated fats are okay to eat. These fats are prevalent in olive oil, canola oil, corn oil, sunflower seed oil, and safflower oil. Go to your cupboard and make certain these oils are there. Next, use them!

Monounsaturated fats like olive and canola oil are especially beneficial because in addition to not contributing to your blood cholesterol, they actually help lower your existing cholesterol! Enjoy that olive oil—in salad dressings, as a bread dip, and for cooking. It's the oil nature intended us to enjoy!

The Bottom Line

Only your physician can determine your ideal saturated fat intake; however, most experts agree on the following figures as a "healthy" amount of saturated fat. These are based on your total calorie consumption.

CALORIES CONSUMED	SATURATED FAT
1,500	12 grams
2,000	16 grams
2,500	19 grams
3,000	23 grams

Count your saturated-fat calories and try to keep them within these figures. Using 7% of your total calories is a good rule of thumb. If you're not eating enough good fat, consider adding an essential fatty acid or omega-3 to your supplement regimen.

TAKE THIS THOUGHT TO BED WITH YOU

You have proven that you're not a quitter, you're a winner. And you're one of the people who will use your stick-to-it-ness to reach all your goals.

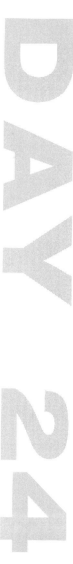

Do it! Write it! Be it!

WHAT YOU ATE (If you swallowed it, write it down)

Breakfast:

Lunch:

Supper:

_____ _____ _____
_____ _____ _____
_____ _____ _____
_____ _____ _____
_____ _____ _____
_____ _____ _____
_____ _____ _____
_____ _____ _____

Snacks:

WHAT YOU DID

Cardiovascular Exercise   Time   Notes

_____ _____ _____
_____ _____ _____

Resistance Exercise   Reps/Sets/Weight   Notes

_____ _____ _____
_____ _____ _____
_____ _____ _____
_____ _____ _____
_____ _____ _____
_____ _____ _____
_____ _____ _____

WHAT YOU THOUGHT

ONLY 4 DAYS TO GO!

DAY 25

BRAIN POWER

There is a tremendous mental and physical capacity that our bodies have that we don't tap into. It is estimated we use less than 30% of our brains, and less than 50% of our physical prowess.

Challenge yourself! When a day gets you down and you don't think you have anything left, reach into those extra reserves—just a bit. Reach into them every time you work out and you'll get more for your time invested. As you use these reserves, your endurance will build and you will feel so much better! The bottom line: If you think you can't, you won't. Always think you can and believe in yourself.

EATING RIGHT

Another healthy eating day. Think fresh. Think whole foods. Think organic. Think natural.

BREAKFAST

Breakfast on the go: Still too rushed to sit down for breakfast? That's life in the fast lane, so thank goodness for all the variety in meal replacement bars, shakes, smoothies, and even soups! Remember, never more than two of your three main meals should be replaced by a supplement bar or shake.

Sit-down breakfast: Sauté diced bell pepper, diced onion, and finely diced broccoli crowns in a pan coated with Pam, then add egg substitute, egg whites or three egg whites with one egg yolk for you yolk-lovers, and scramble them alongside the vegetables. Enjoy the scramble with half a cantaloupe and two slices of rye or pumpernickel bread with almond butter. Enjoy your coffee, tea, or nonfat milk on the side.

LUNCH

Lunch on the go: Have soup and salad at a deli or sandwich bar that makes home-made soups. Avoid cream-based soups in favor of broth-based soups. Use no more than two tablespoons of dressing on your salad. Drink plenty of water.

Sit-down lunch: Make it a soup-and-salad day! Seek out bean, lentil, or pea soup. Make it from scratch, a soup starter, or out of the can. Always seek out low-sodium canned soups such as Healthy Choice. Use low- or nonfat dressing and no more than two tablespoons on your green and leafy salad. Have fruit for dessert and drink at least eight ounces of water.

SUPPER

Supper on the go: A meal replacement shake or smoothie with fresh fruit. Have a handful of raw mixed nuts and a low-fat, low-sugar yogurt, preferably plain. Drink lots of water and snack on celery and carrot sticks.

Sit-down supper: Have you had your fish today? Try a salmon steak, mahi-mahi, sole, or swordfish, broiled in the oven or on a George Foreman grill. Add a cup of wild rice and a medley of mixed green, orange, and yellow vegetables (broccoli, carrots, yellow peppers) with mushrooms, lightly stir-fried in a tablespoon of olive oil.

Always drink plenty of water with your meals. A diet soda is in order tonight if you prefer.

WORKOUT

We're back to hitting the cardio and the abs again.

CARDIOVASCULAR EXERCISE

Pick your form of cardio: walking, marching, stair climbing, gliding, exercising on the treadmill, cycling, or aerobic dancing. Go for the burn, go for the interval, and go for a bonus five minutes today. Go for 30 to 45 minutes of continuous, non-stop, fat-burning exercise!

Remember your Two-Minute Warning, and go for it! Then cool down for three to five minutes, until your heart rate is 100 or under.

1. Reverse crunch (lower abdominals):

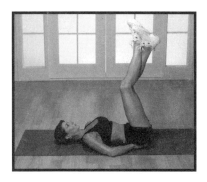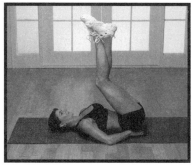

For at home or at the gym. Think *squeeze* and technique! Don't let that lower back come too far off the ground, and breathe out as you bear down on the lower abs.

SET ONE: 10–15 repetitions
SET TWO: 10–15 repetitions
SET THREE: 10–15 repetitions

2. Oblique crunch (abdominals):

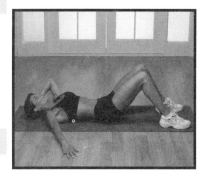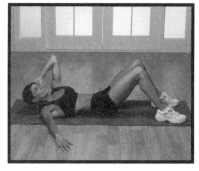

This move works both the abs and the obliques. Lie on a pad. Without pulling your head forward and with your chin up, pull your left elbow and shoulder toward your right knee and *squeeze*. Alternate with your right elbow and shoulder pulling toward your left knee.

SET ONE: 10–25 repetitions
SET TWO: 10–25 repetitions
SET THREE: 10–25 repetitions

3. Lying back extension (lower back):

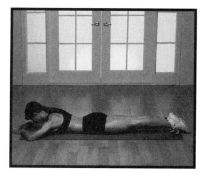 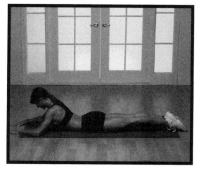

For at home or at the gym. Push up in a smooth, fluid motion. Try to keep your back straight and your neck neutral throughout.

SET ONE: 10–15 repetitions
SET TWO: 10–15 repetitions

HEALTH SMARTS

DRINK TEA TO ENHANCE YOUR HEALTH

Next to plain water, tea is the most consumed beverage in the world. In the United Kingdom, the average person drinks three or four cups of tea a day. Tea is touted with having myriad health benefits, including substantial antioxidant activity that may combat heart disease and cancer.

Drinking certain teas has been said to reduce serum cholesterol levels, lower blood pressure, and even slow the aging process. Two types of tea have had a recent surge in popularity in the United States, and are the subject of numerous scientific studies: green tea and black tea.

There are only three types of tea—green tea, black tea, and oolong tea—but there are some 3,000 variations of these types. All tea is derived from the Camellia sinensis tree. Some herbs, like chamomile, are incorrectly referred to as tea. Herbal "teas" normally contain flowers, leaves, and ingredients from a variety of different plants, and are not true teas by definition. Just remember not to overdo the tea at the expense of water. Water is more hydrating than tea.

Green tea: Green tea is a light, refreshing tea that's fast becoming known as a "functional food" because it appears to have several bio-regulating properties. Green tea's special benefits are claimed to be fortification of the immune system, disease prevention (such as preventing high blood pressure), disease recovery (such as inhibiting the rise of cholesterol), and anti-aging (due to its antioxidant action).

Antioxidants prevent cellular damage caused by harmful free radicals in our body that can lead to diseases like cancer.

Most researchers believe that the health benefits of tea come from a family of nutrients called polyphenols. In green tea, substances called catechins make up the largest percentage of polyphenols.

According to one study at the University of Texas in 1997, green tea contains "the strongest of any known form of antioxidants." The study found that the catechin content in green tea was "more than 100 times as effective at neutralizing free radicals as Vitamin C, and 25 times more powerful than Vitamin E."

Black tea: Black tea accounts for about 70% of the world's tea consumption. Black tea has a much heartier taste and a deeper color than green tea. The most popular types of black tea are English breakfast, Irish breakfast, Darjeeling, Ceylon, and orange pekoe. Since black tea is oxidized (or "fermented"), most of the beneficial catechins are destroyed. However, black tea contains other antioxidants called flavonoids.

Black tea contains many essential vitamins and minerals, including Vitamin B_1 (thiamin), B_2 (riboflavin) and B_6, folic acid, calcium, manganese, potassium, and zinc. Also, both black and green teas are natural sources of fluoride, which helps prevent cavities.

Handy tea tips: To make the perfect cup of tea, bring fresh water to a full boil. Using one tea bag for each cup, pour boiling water over the bag and let it steep. Green tea needs to steep for about two to three minutes; black tea should steep for about five minutes, or longer if you like it strong. Green tea is best when served plain, or with an orange slice or a dash of nutmeg for variety. The most popular way to drink black tea is with some milk, and a sugar substitute if you like it sweet.

According to the Lipton Company, tea bags don't lose their antioxidant potency if they've been sitting around for a long time. However, old tea can have a stale taste.

Iced tea was invented in the United States. After tea is brewed, it retains about 80% of its antioxidants for the next 48 hours. For food safety reasons, do not store iced tea for longer than 48 hours and always store it in the refrigerator.

Tea contains much less caffeine than regular coffee, and also less than some colas. Brewed coffee contains about 120 mg. of caffeine in a six-ounce cup. For the same six ounces, black tea contains around 40 mg., and green tea around 30 mg. of caffeine.

An ancient Chinese monk named Eisai once said, "Tea is a miraculous medicine for the maintenance of health. Tea has an extraordinary power to prolong life. Anywhere a person cultivates tea, long life will follow." Today, Western science is just starting to unveil the powerful health benefits of tea that Asian cultures have understood for centuries.

TAKE THIS THOUGHT TO BED WITH YOU

You've had another big day, so you need a good night's rest. Then get up in the morning and kick butt!

Do it! Write it! Be it!

WHAT YOU ATE (If you swallowed it, write it down)

Breakfast: Lunch: Supper:

_____ _____ _____

_____ _____ _____

_____ _____ _____

_____ _____ _____

_____ _____ _____

_____ _____ _____

Snacks:

WHAT YOU DID

Cardiovascular Exercise   Time   Notes

_____ _____ _____

_____ _____ _____

_____ _____ _____

Abdominal Exercise   Rep/Sets   Notes

_____ _____ _____

_____ _____ _____

Other Activities

_____

_____

_____

DAY 25

SUCCESS LOG

WHAT YOU THOUGHT

ONLY 3 DAYS TO GO!

DAY 26

BRAIN POWER

Energy is life. It gives you power, drive, ambition. Eating well and exercising daily will help keep those energy levels up in you. Never, ever give up. Just reach deeper and you will always find what you need inside you. Even if your energy furnace gets low, stoke the fire and get yourself moving again. Once you get the hang of it, you won't be able to stop. Eating the right foods gives you energy.

EATING RIGHT

Good food choices should be like second nature by now. That's the way it's supposed to be. Are you fitting into those tight pants that refused to zip up just three weeks ago? Good job! You must be making good choices.

BREAKFAST

Breakfast on the go: Have some Kashi brand high-fiber cereal with nonfat milk and a piece of fruit or a meal replacement bar or high-protein, low-carb smoothie.

Sit-down breakfast: Mix a scoop of protein powder with low-fat, low-sugar yogurt, preferably plain, berries, fruits, and nuts. Have two slices of whole-grain or rye bread with butter, almond butter or a trans-fat-free spread. Drink a cup of coffee or tea, no sugar, black or with a low-fat cream substitute.

LUNCH

Lunch on the go: Pick up a deli-made tuna salad with lots of greens and not more than two tablespoons of dressing. Some delis prepare their tuna with low-fat mayonnaise.

Sit-down lunch: Have one fist-sized lean hamburger patty, turkey patty, or low-fat veggie burger cooked on a George Foreman grill or fried with Pam. (For added flavor, dip it in A-1 sauce or ketchup.) On the side have a slice of avocado, cottage cheese, and warm black or kidney beans.

Have an apple or orange for dessert. Drink at least eight ounces of water.

SUPPER

Supper on the go: Grab a meal replacement shake with extra fresh fruit and a handful of unsalted walnuts and almonds, plus lots of water.

Sit-down supper: Grill or bake your choice of flank steak, sole, or tofu scramble or patties. Add a fist-sized portion of a green vegetable, or salad with oil and vinegar, fat-free Italian dressing, or balsamic vinegar. Enjoy one cup of rice; wild is preferred, but brown or white will do. Go easy on the soy sauce. And don't ever, ever forget to drink plenty of water.

WORKOUT

Feeling muscles you never knew you had before? During today's workout try to really get in touch with your muscles. If you have a mirror, perform the exercises in front of it and really watch the muscles work. Direct 100% of your mental energy right to that muscle group.

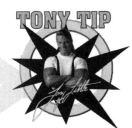

Never sleepwalk through an exercise. Pay attention, check your log to see what you did during the workouts in the past, then push for a bit more. Concentrate on the muscle, on technique, and on squeezing the muscle worked and the surrounding supportive muscles—especially the abs—throughout the movement.

CARDIOVASCULAR EXERCISE

Here we go again. Invest 40 minutes of your time. Remember to work at a PRE (Perceived Rate of Exertion) of 6 to 8. Be sure to keep track of everything in your logbooks!

RESISTANCE EXERCISE

Okay. Muster up some energy for one more killer calorie-burning workout, then you'll have two days of rest. You can do it. It's your last workout of the week!

And cut me some slack. I took out the ab exercises today so you can really put in a calorie-burning, lean muscle-building workout!

> **Note:** Challenge yourself, but keep exercise form!

1. **Full squat** (front and back of upper legs and butt):

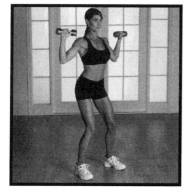 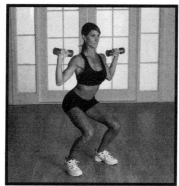

For at home or at the gym. Holding two dumbbells (as shown), stand with your feet shoulder-width apart. Now slowly lower yourself as if you were about to sit in a chair. Go as far down as you're comfortable, ideally until your thighs are parallel to the floor. Squeeze your thighs and butt on the way up.

SET ONE: 10–15 repetitions
SET TWO: 10–15 repetitions
SET THREE: 10–15 repetitions

1a. Leg press machine (front of upper legs and butt):

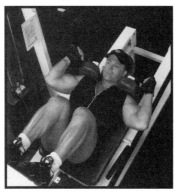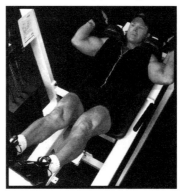

For the gym only. Position the machine so that your knees are bent and you're a little squished at the start. The first portion of this exercise hits the glutes and creates a great looking butt! Push your legs out until they are straight, but don't lock the knees. Then return, under control, to the start. Machines vary, so experiment with the poundage. You might be a lot stronger on this than you think!

SET ONE: 10–15 repetitions
SET TWO: 10–15 repetitions
SET THREE: 10–15 repetitions

2. Stationary lunge (hamstrings, gluteals):

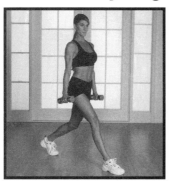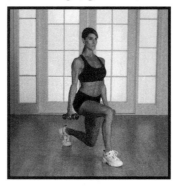

For at home or at the gym. Hold dumbbells in each hand. Perform this lunge by standing upright and taking a large stride forward with your right leg. This is the start position. Let your left knee trail as low as is comfortable. Keep your forward knee over the ball of your foot. Stand back up to the start position—think squeeze. Finish all your reps for one leg before moving to the other leg.

SET ONE: 8–10 repetitions
SET TWO: 8–10 repetitions
SET THREE: 8–10 repetitions

2a. Leg extension (quadriceps):

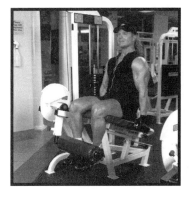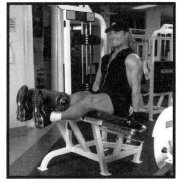

For the gym only. Hold onto the side handles. Squeeze your quads as you extend your legs straight out in front of you. Hold for one second at the peak contraction, then lower the bar.

SET ONE: 10–15 repetitions
SET TWO: 10–15 repetitions
SET THREE: 10–15 repetitions

3. Wide-stance squat (legs, inner thighs):

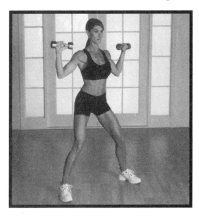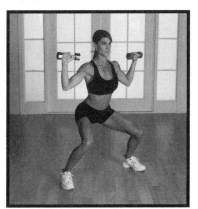

For at home or at the gym. Hold dumbbells as shown. Stand with your feet wider apart than shoulder width, toes pointed out at ten and two o'clock. Keep your back straight and eyes up and squat down as far as comfortable and *squeeze* your glutes!

SET ONE: 10–15 repetitions
SET TWO: 10–15 repetitions
SET THREE: 10–15 repetitions

3a. Leg press machine (quads, gluteals):

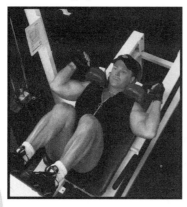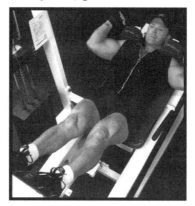

For the gym only. Begin by pushing the platform up past the slide guards. Once you remove these guards, the machine has the capability to come nearly all the way down. Be certain the weight is under your control. With abs, arms, and legs tense, lower the weight as far as comfortable and without reversing the motion. Squeeze back to the top.

> **SET ONE:** 10-15 repetitions
> **SET TWO:** 10-15 repetitions
> **SET THREE:** 10-15 repetitions

4. Back Row with chair (v-taper of back):

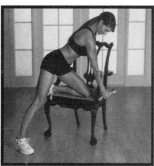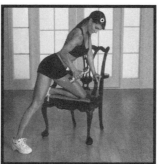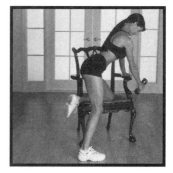

For at home or at the gym. This is a great exercise for strengthening the back. At home, find a sturdy armless chair and kneel on it as shown. In the gym, use a bench. Try and keep your chest almost parallel to the floor and your back straight, balance on the chair with one arm and hold a dumbbell (use a light, 5- to 20-pound dumbbell) at arm's length in the other hand. Keeping your upper body tense, squeeze the dumbbell up to the side of your chest, elbow slightly bent out, then return to arm's length and stretch (but not to the floor).

SET ONE: 10–15 repetitions
SET TWO: 10–15 repetitions
SET THREE: 10–15 repetitions

4a. Back row machine (back):

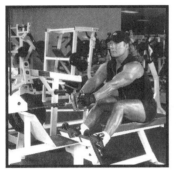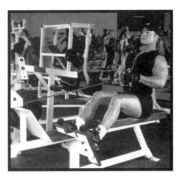

For the gym only. Grab the close-grip handles on a rowing machine with a 45-degree back, then push back with your legs until there is tension on the cable. From this position, pull the handles close to your body and squeeze your shoulder blades at the peak of the movement. Return to the original position.

SET ONE: 10–15 repetitions
SET TWO: 10–15 repetitions
SET THREE: 10–15 repetitions

5. Reverse grip shoulder press (shoulders):

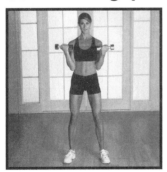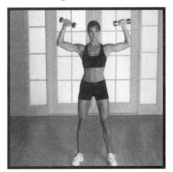

For at home or at the gym. With knees slightly bent, stand with your feet shoulder-width apart. Holding a dumbbell in each hand, palms facing toward your body in a reverse grip, pull the dumbbells up to your shoulders. Then press up, rotating so your palms face away from your body at the peak of the movement. Return to the original position.

Avoid the tendency to arch your back and look up while performing this exercise. If you have trouble maintaining correct posture, you're probably using weights that are too heavy. In the gym you can use a special bench to support your back or use a shoulder press machine.

SET ONE: 10–15 repetitions
SET TWO: 10–15 repetitions
SET THREE: 10–15 repetitions

5a. Upright cable row (for upper shoulders, neck):

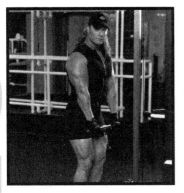 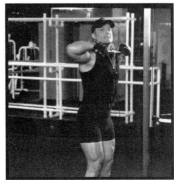

For the gym only. Begin by facing a low pulley with a short bar. Bend down and pull it to arms' length. Bending your elbows, squeeze the bar up under your chin. Bring your elbows as high as possible and really squeeze on the trapezius muscles that run across the top of your shoulders. Lower under control.

SET ONE: 10–15 repetitions
SET TWO: 10–15 repetitions
SET THREE: 10–15 repetitions

6. Side lateral (shoulders):

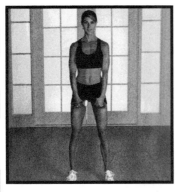 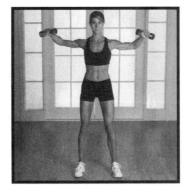

For at home or at the gym. Stand with your feet shoulder-width apart and hold a dumbbell in each hand at arms' length. In an arc, bring the dumbbells up and *squeeze*. Keep your elbows slightly bent throughout the movement.

SET ONE: 10–12 repetitions
SET TWO: 10–12 repetitions
SET THREE: 10–12 repetitions

6a. Lateral cable raise (shoulders):

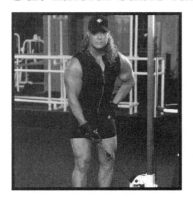 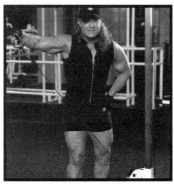

For the gym only. Begin standing alongside a low cable with a single handle. Pick up the handle and stand erect. In a fluid motion, raise the cable out away from your body and squeeze to shoulder height. Pause, then return.

SET ONE: 10–12 repetitions
SET TWO: 10–12 repetitions
SET THREE: 10–12 repetitions

7. Concentration curl (biceps):

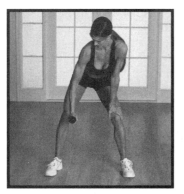 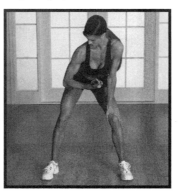

For at home or at the gym. Rest one hand inside your knee for stability, and hold the dumbbell palm up in the other hand. Really concentrate on squeezing your biceps.

SET ONE: 10–15 repetitions
SET TWO: 10–15 repetitions
SET THREE: 10–15 repetitions

7a. Arm curl machine or preacher bench (biceps):

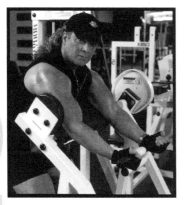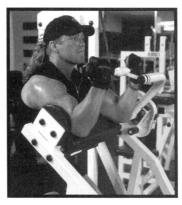

For the gym only. Adjust the set so you can hold the handles at arms' length. Squeezing hard on your biceps, curl the handles up as high as possible. Hold and really squeeze for the peak contraction. Don't use heavy weight on this exercise.

SET ONE: 10–15 repetitions
SET TWO: 10–15 repetitions
SET THREE: 10–15 repetitions

8. Triceps kickback (triceps):

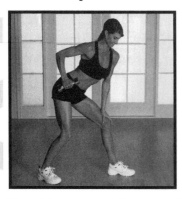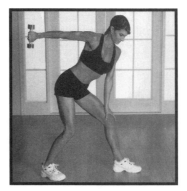

For at home or at the gym. With a dumbbell at arm's length at your side, bend at the elbow and bring your upper arm up so that it is level with your back. This is the start position. Do not move that upper arm! To perform, simply "kick back" and *squeeze* your hand and forearm so you arm is straight. Really put the squeeze on the triceps throughout the movement!

SET ONE: 10–12 repetitions
SET TWO: 10–12 repetitions
SET THREE: 10–12 repetitions

8a. Seated triceps extension (triceps):

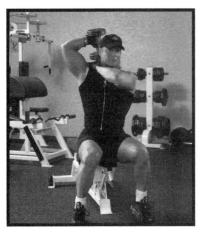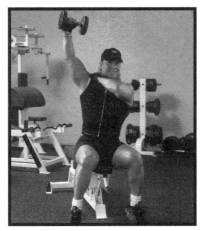

For the gym only. Sit at the end of a bench and hold a dumbbell (as shown) behind your head. Use your other arm to help stabilize the lifting arm and keep the upper arm in the same position as you raise the dumbbell to arms' length and *squeeze*.

SET ONE: 10–12 repetitions
SET TWO: 10–12 repetitions
SET THREE: 10–12 repetitions

Finish off with some light stretching. Walking around will loosen up those leg muscles!

HEALTH SMARTS

CRAVINGS

Men's cravings for meat and high-protein foods and women's cravings for sweets and chocolate in particular are instinctual. We crave the foods we need for survival. In some ways, we may have been better off left to our instincts.

We are designed to crave foods that contain the vital nutrients—fat, protein, and carbohydrates—that our bodies need to survive. While you may not intellectually realize that strawberries are a great source of Vitamin C, if you were Vitamin C deficient and someone passed a plump ripe strawberry under your nose, you'd perk up like the dog when he hears you pick up his food bowl.

In prehistoric times, for women to procreate they needed to have enough stored fat to survive nine months of near-famine times with enough left over to give birth to a healthy baby and then breast-feed it. Nature built into women cravings for foods that will be stored as fat. Anthropologists surmise that because these foods were rare, humans learned to identify them and seek them out. Over thousands of years, this adaptation has become a permanent part of a woman's biochemical makeup.

Chocolate's Secret Ingredient

It's not that women crave chocolate, but that they crave nutrients that stimulate serotonin. A leading authority, Dr. Margaret Pranger, refers to serotonin as the "happy chemical" for women.

"When we are depressed or upset, we [women] crave serotonin," says Pranger. "And part of PMS is low serotonin. This is the way it works: women crave serotonin. Foods that stimulate serotonin are high-glycemic. High-glycemic foods stimulate our main fat-storing enzyme, lipoprotein lipase. High-glycemic foods elevate serotonin and make us fatter."

Men have cravings too, but they tend toward high protein. Thus, couples go to fast-food restaurants (and other places), with the man seeking meat and the woman seeking high-glycemic foods. They share the meal of meat, potatoes, and dessert and each leaves satisfied, each in their own way.

The problem is that our hardwiring that tells us to grab available nutrients at every chance we get is no longer valid. The human body didn't know we would someday have fast-food restaurants at every corner and grocery shelves filled with high-glycemic breads and pastas and more. We still crave, but we crave over and above what anyone would need for simple survival.

You can't teach an old body new tricks overnight. But you can work toward providing your body with an optimum level of macronutrients so you don't instigate cravings. For men, that usually means additional protein. For women, that means low-glycemic carbohydrates, as recommended in this program.

TAKE THIS THOUGHT TO BED WITH YOU

You've had a big day and a long workout. Treat yourself to a warm bath, Jacuzzi, or back rub. You deserve it. Then just kick back and relax. Good workout! Good night!

Do it! Write it! Be it!

WHAT YOU ATE (If you swallowed it, write it down)

Breakfast: Lunch: Supper:

_____   _____   _____
_____   _____   _____
_____   _____   _____
_____   _____   _____
_____   _____   _____
_____   _____   _____
_____   _____   _____

Snacks:

WHAT YOU DID

Cardiovascular Exercise	Time	Notes
_____	_____	_____
_____	_____	_____

Resistance Exercise	Reps/Sets/Weight	Notes
_____	_____	_____
_____	_____	_____
_____	_____	_____
_____	_____	_____
_____	_____	_____
_____	_____	_____

WHAT YOU THOUGHT

_____
_____
_____
_____
_____
_____
_____
_____
_____
_____
_____
_____
_____
_____
_____
_____
_____
_____
_____
_____
_____
_____
_____
_____
_____
_____
_____
_____
_____
_____
_____
_____

ONLY 2 DAYS TO GO!

DAY 27

BRAIN POWER

Life will pass you by if you give it the chance, so don't let it. Nobody has ever won big on a sure bet. Take your chances and go for the most out of your life. Constantly keep your mind looking toward new goals and new aspirations and be sure to take the necessary actions to achieve them. A youthful attitude and its excitement are not the products of time, they are products of the mind. Don't let them slip away.

EATING RIGHT

By now, some of your bad habits must be gone and replaced by a few good ones, like having smaller portions, more little meals, less sugar, more water, and more protein. This in itself is going to go a long way in making you look and feel better.

BREAKFAST

Breakfast on the go: Grab a meal replacement bar or drink, some fresh fruit, and a bottle of water as you head out the door!

Sit-down breakfast: Try half a cup of slow-cooked oats (or low-fat, low-sodium, high-fiber cereal) with berries, nuts, and nonfat milk. Or, have a scoop of protein powder mixed with low-fat, low-sugar yogurt, preferably plain. Also have a slice of whole-grain bread with butter or a trans-fat-free spread. Drink a cup of coffee or tea, no sugar, black or with a low-fat cream substitute.

You're loaded with high-energy carbohydrates and slow-burning protein, so head out the door, full steam ahead!

LUNCH

Lunch on the go: Try one of Subway's six-inch, under-six-grams-of-fat sandwiches or a healthy meal replacement. Don't forget the water! Or, go to a deli and ask them to make you a sandwich, light on the mayonnaise!

Sit-down lunch: Make a couple of bean burritos with extra lettuce or go out for a chunky chicken salad, fajita salad, or Cobb salad without the bacon. Keep dressings on the side and use no more than two tablespoons.

SUPPER

Supper on the go: Grab a fist-sized portion of lean meat from the deli and enjoy with a cup of lentil or split pea soup, or a three-bean or pasta salad. Enjoy a low-fat, low-sugar yogurt, preferably plain, with nuts or fresh fruit for dessert, and water.

Sit-down supper: Indulge yourself with a generous fist-sized lean meat or other protein source, plus a fist-sized portion of vegetables and low-glycemic carbohydrates. Finish with a low-fat, low-sugar yogurt, preferably plain, mixed with nuts and your favorite fruit. Don't forget to drink plenty of water.

WORKOUT

Today's another day of active rest/cardio and abs.

CARDIOVASCULAR EXERCISE

Pick your favorite cardio activity, or find an activity to keep you moving, nonstop, for 30 to 45 minutes.

RESISTANCE EXERCISE

We're skipping resistance today, but I'd like you to perform a quick set of ab crunches and some more side twists to keep that lower back limber.

1. Side twist (trunk, lower back):

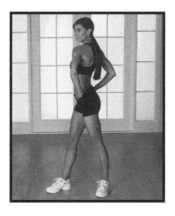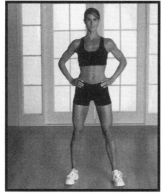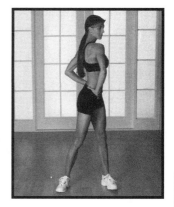

For at home. Stand with your feet shoulder-width apart, hands on your hips. Keep your shoulders still, and use the muscles below your waist to twist or swivel your hips in a fluid motion to the right, center and left. The three positions constitute one rep.

> **SET ONE:** 10–20 repetitions each direction
> **SET TWO:** 10–20 repetitions each direction

2. Ab crunch (upper abdominals):

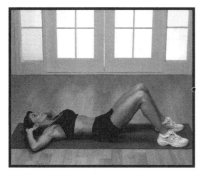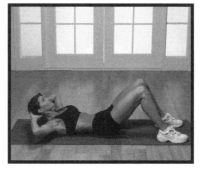

For at home. Use 100% of your concentration to keep your body as tense as possible and to keep these movements slow and precise. Think *squeeze* and technique!

> **SET ONE:** 10–15 repetitions
> **SET TWO:** 10–15 repetitions
> **SET THREE:** 10–15 repetitions

DAY 27

3. Reverse crunch (lower abdominals):

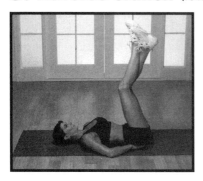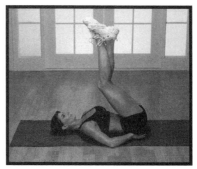

For at home. Think technique! Keep your knees pressed together and really bear down on those lower abs. Feel the muscle and use the *squeeze* technique!

SET ONE: 10–15 repetitions
SET TWO: 10–15 repetitions
SET THREE: 10–15 repetitions

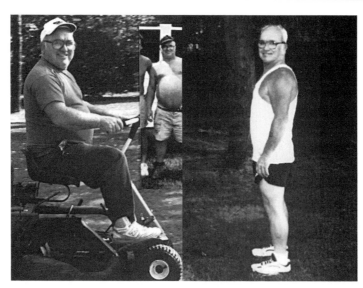

The proof is in the success stories of millions like yourself. Meet John Bradford from Maryland who lost 73 pounds following the "Tony Way." We're very proud of him!

A LITTLE HELP FROM YOUR FRIENDS: THE VALUE OF PERSONAL TRAINERS

Personal trainers can get you results that are very difficult, if not impossible, to achieve on your own. Now that you've almost come to the end of my one-on-one program, you might consider a personal trainer to keep you on track.

There are five primary things a personal trainer should do for you:

1. Assessment: Your personal trainer should spend the first session assessing your base level of strength, your flexibility, and any preexisting injuries or limitations you may have. The trainer should then ask you an extensive set of questions to ascertain your short- and long-term goals and then make a mutually agreed upon list. At your next session, you should expect a routine written specifically for your goals.

2. Commitment: Your trainer should have you sign an agreement and make a financial commitment for a certain number of weeks. Nothing short of a medical excuse (with a note from the doctor!) should excuse you from a workout.

3. Encouragement: Your trainer should provide you with his or her full attention and provide you with plenty of encouragement. Keeping track of each of your accomplishments and personal bests is a great way to keep you pushing harder. Your trainer should be teaching you the joy of working out. This isn't all laughter and chitchat. It's about learning to push yourself harder on each repetition, and allowing yourself to bask in the glory when you know you've put your all into an activity.

4. Objectivity: The one thing you can rarely do on your own is objectively decide when your condition is optimum. You may have wanted to lose 20 pounds, but after the first 20 you got so excited you dropped below a healthy weight. You may have always wanted to see your abdominal muscles, but never noticed the rest of your body was out of balance. A good trainer should be able to guide you toward a better body than the one you've anticipated.

5. Goal Revision: As you progress with a personal trainer, he or she should stay on top of your goals, remind you when you've reached them, and then help you formulate new goals. The trainer should always keep you goal-conscious. Seeing the end (a new, in-shape body) is important to sticking with the process.

I love personal trainers with enthusiasm and great motivational techniques.

One of the best things a trainer can do is to keep you focused on your workouts. Total concentration while working out is necessary to see fast results. Gum chewing, reading books on the cardio machines, and even watching TV takes your attention away from the task at hand. This is where a good trainer can dial you into your workouts, let you rejoice in the feeling of your body working hard and start you on a path of lifelong fitness.

Remember, time is precious.
Make every minute count.

TAKE THIS THOUGHT TO BED WITH YOU

Tomorrow is the last day of the program, and the first day of your new life. You've got decisions to make. Start thinking of where you want to bring your fitness—how far you want to go. Our personal training hotlines at 1-800-780-6744 are there to help you with the means to accomplish any and all of your health and fitness goals.

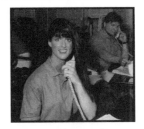

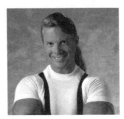

Do it! Write it! Be it!

WHAT YOU ATE (If you swallowed it, write it down)

Breakfast: Lunch: Supper:

_____   _____   _____

_____   _____   _____

_____   _____   _____

_____   _____   _____

_____   _____   _____

_____   _____   _____

_____   _____   _____

Snacks:

WHAT YOU DID

Cardiovascular Exercise   Time   Notes

_____   _____   _____

_____   _____   _____

_____   _____   _____

_____   _____   _____

Ab Work   Sets   Notes

_____   _____   _____

_____   _____   _____

_____   _____   _____

Other Activities

_____

_____

_____

DAY 27 SUCCESS LOG

WHAT YOU THOUGHT

_____
_____
_____
_____
_____
_____
_____
_____
_____
_____
_____
_____
_____
_____
_____
_____
_____
_____
_____
_____
_____
_____
_____
_____
_____
_____
_____
_____
_____
_____

ONLY 1 DAY TO GO!

DAY 28

BRAIN POWER

Sundays are often days of reflection. How appropriate it is that we end on a day on which we can take some time and look closely back at the last four weeks. Read your training logs and remember how the process began, progressed, and ultimately changed you.

Are you emotionally stronger? Do you have a better outlook? More energy? Fewer sleepless nights? Are you happier? Thinner? Standing taller? Looking better than you did four weeks ago? Sure, all of those are true. That's the beauty of good nutrition and proper exercise. Keep them in your daily life, forever.

EATING RIGHT

Remember to have at every meal water, protein, low-glycemic carbohydrates, and small portions.

BREAKFAST

Breakfast on the go: Reach for a high-protein, low-carbohydrate meal replacement smoothie or bar. Remember to drink at least eight ounces of water with breakfast, and don't forget a multiple vitamin/mineral supplement.

Sit-down breakfast: Have three eggs (or egg substitute), poached, fried with Pam spray, or scrambled. On the side, have two slices of sourdough or rye bread with I Can't Believe It's Not Butter spray or a trans-fat-free spread. Drink one cup of coffee or tea, no sugar, black or with a low-fat cream substitute. You may also have a six-ounce glass of orange juice or apple juice, or a piece of fruit. Try to eat the fruit or bread before the eggs, if possible. Don't forget a daily multiple vitamin/mineral supplement every morning!

Now enjoy a great day because you've got plenty of high-octane fuel!

LUNCH

Lunch on the go: Grab that high-protein, low-carbohydrate meal replacement smoothie or bar. Be sure to drink plenty of water with lunch and throughout the day!

Restrict your on-the-go meal replacement bars to no more than two a day. You may choose ready-to-drink smoothies and shakes and keep a stockpile in your fridge. Or, you may mix your own with ice, water or nonfat milk and a high-protein, low-carbohydrate powder with frozen strawberries.

Sit-down lunch: Add a small amount of low-fat mayonnaise or Miracle Whip to a six- or eight-ounce can of water-packed tuna. Mix with peas and/or chopped celery and spread onto two slices of whole-grain, sourdough, rye, or pumpernickel bread for a high-protein, low-carbohydrate lunch. Hint: add a little mustard or pickle relish to moisten your tuna salad.

If you don't like tuna, try a chicken breast—grilled, baked, or broiled without the skin—on two slices of bread with lettuce, tomato, and mayonnaise. Turkey is also okay as long as it's breast meat.

Have an apple or orange for dessert. Drink at least eight ounces of water.

SUPPER

Supper on the go: Drink a high-protein, low-carbohydrate smoothie or shake, or eat one high-protein, low-carbohydrate bar. Remember, never exceed two meal replacements per day; you need to have at least one sit-down meal a day!

Be sure to drink eight ounces or more of water with your meal replacement!

Sit-down supper: Grill or broil a two- to three-ounce cube steak patty (you may substitute tuna steak, salmon, chicken breast, or turkey), and add a fist-sized portion of green beans, lima beans, spinach, or salad with oil and vinegar, fat-free Italian dressing, or balsamic vinegar. Have a sweet or baked potato with light butter or trans-fat-free spread (read the label). Try a bit of A-1 sauce on your potato—it tastes great!

Again, drink plenty of water. Water helps you lose body fat and it's great for your skin.

WORKOUT

Congratulations! You've made it through! What you have just completed is a serious program aimed at changing habits that have taken a lifetime to develop. These habits contributed to your weight gain, sluggishness, lack of self-esteem, or other factors that drove you to try this program.

You don't need to perform any formal exercise today, but why don't you treat yourself to a party—even if it's a party of one? Get outside, weather permitting, and enjoy the world we live in. Turn up some music and dance or sing along with some of your favorites. Take yourself shopping—you may need some new clothes! Or just curl up with a good book—as long as you promise every third chapter you'll get up and move around for about ten minutes.

Enjoy this day off and use it for reflection on how far you have come.

Your Future

Now it's time to get a gym membership or hire a personal trainer. For more information and exercises, you can also go to my website (www.tonylittle. com) or call my personal training hotline at 1-800-780-6744.

It's now up to you to keep the momentum going and make the habits you've developed a lifestyle for longevity!

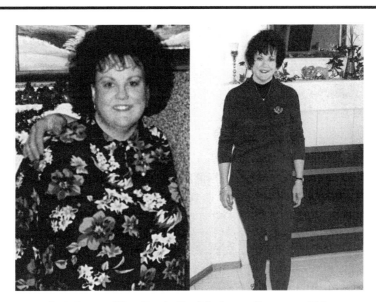

Celebrate like Beth Smith from Oregon did
when she lost 100 pounds.
She did it! And so can you!

READING BETWEEN THE LINES

News hounds peruse medical journals daily in search of health-related headlines. Headlines draw the reader into the story, which nearly always requires some sensationalizing. And reporters love to find medical studies from which they can dissect one tiny element and banner it to the world as if it were gospel.

Thus, while we are far better informed now about health and nutrition than at any other time, we are also more confused. Should we eat more fat? Is a little exercise as good as a lot? Are carbohydrates evil? If you take the news at face value you probably can't answer any of those questions!

On one particular day, the following appeared on the newsstands simultaneously:

▶ "It's now considered O.K. to put on a few pounds in your senior years . . . finds a study."—*The New York Times*
▶ "This week's *New England Journal of Medicine* provides the best evidence yet that extra weight is unhealthy."—*USA Today*
▶ "A new study shows obesity poses less threat than thought."—*Time*

The source of all three was a study of 320,000 healthy, nonsmoking white adults who were tracked for 12 years. The researchers used the Body Mass Index (BMI) to measure their body fat and then computed the age-related death rates for various degrees of being overweight.

The study found that being overweight was linked to higher death rates, especially from cardiovascular disease, up to age 75. After age 75, death rates did not increase with having extra weight.

The study found the greatest risk was in young people who were very overweight and that extra weight was slightly more dangerous for men than for women. However, it takes a stretch of the imagination to figure how the *Time* editors came up with their headline in light of the study's findings.

I'm sure plenty of overweight people read the *Time* headline only, and then went back for seconds on the cheesecake. We all tend to hear what we want to hear. Sometimes you have to play the devil's advocate, and question studies that say a little bit of walking is all you need. If that was all it took, why would so many people want—and need—so much to look and feel their best?

When reading about a study, dig to find the numbers. How many subjects were involved in the study? The more the better. Who conducted the study? An academic institution or a drug manufacturer? How long was the study conducted for? The longer the better. If you have a study of more than 500,000 participants, conducted by a school or research institute and for a duration of at least ten years, you probably have some valid data to peruse.

Don't read what you want to read into the headlines. The one irrefutable fact about American health is that being overweight can kill.

Listen to your body. Follow your instincts. You've learned how good you can feel by exercising and eating healthy. Never forget that. And when you feel sluggish and achy and without any energy, look to see if you've slacked up on some of the components of good health you've learned in this program. Better yet, start again from day one.

It's the process that counts. You've learned the talk and the walk. Now put them into motion to stay on the right track to a long, healthy, vital lifetime.

MEASURING YOUR PROGRESS

You should have been periodically checking your measurements all along, and have probably seen quite a difference from the first day. Now, on your last day, take a few minutes to measure the areas marked and compare how far you've come from the first day. I am sure you will find a significant difference because of all the hard work you have put into your health and fitness. Congratulations!

ON OUR LAST NIGHT

Take this book to bed with you tonight. Go back and read each of your 28 daily logs. Highlight the important points you want to remember and use them in your everyday, high-energy, self-confident lifestyle. If you haven't made as much progress as you'd like, look at the effort you put in and see if you could pump up your efforts. Read between the lines to find the days you were really focused, and the days that were ho-hum. Try to understand what made the difference and make all your days ahead better and more productive.

As we've reached the end, you've got to admit it, you're gonna miss me a little bit, right? Well, you may not miss me, but you would miss the workouts. So, it's okay to repeat the last two weeks several times. Or, pick a week and stick with it for a month. Your exercise program doesn't end with this book. It's up to you to keep it going!

You are a winner. You've proved that by making it this far.

ONE FINAL THOUGHT

Life is not measured by the breaths we take, but by the moments that take our breath away. Protect, cherish, and nurture your own good health to give you and your loved ones more of those moments.

Congratulations! You took charge of your life!

God bless you and good night,

Tony Little

Do it! Write it! Be it!

WHAT YOU ATE (If you swallowed it, write it down)

Breakfast: Lunch: Supper:

_____   _____   _____

Snacks:

WHAT YOU DID

Cardiovascular Exercise   Time   Notes

_____   _____   _____

HOW YOU REWARDED YOURSELF

WHAT YOU THOUGHT

Tomorrow is the first day of the rest of your healthy, fit, and fabulous life!

APPENDIX ONE
Stretching

STRETCHING IS LIKE oiling your joints and other moving parts. The benefits of stretching go beyond simply increasing flexibility. Stretching can make you feel more relaxed by reducing muscle tension. It can also prevent muscle strains, promote circulation, and prevent and even cure certain types of back pain. If that's not enough, how about the fact that stretching feels good and takes only a few minutes a day?

For best results, perform a warm-up prior to stretching, such as five to ten minutes of low-intensity aerobic activity. Doing so will raise the body temperature and enable you to stretch farther. You should stretch in loose, comfortable clothing and without any jewelry on. A nonskid, firm mat is ideal for stretching, and the area you're stretching in should be quiet so you can concentrate. Finally, although stretching can be performed anywhere and anytime, it's probably not a good idea to stretch immediately after eating.

It's also beneficial to stretch after a workout, when the muscles are warm. However, they are also contracted after a workout, and you will need to ease slowly into the stretch. It may take a little longer, 15 to 20 minutes, but your muscles will be happier for the effort.

There are many excellent books available on stretching, and if you're interested in pursuing this subject in greater detail, check out Michael J. Alter's *Sport Stretch* (Human Kinetics) and Bob Anderson's *Stretching* (Shelter Publications). For now, here are a few guidelines that most experts agree upon:

1. Stretch slowly, moving smoothly into each stretch.
2. Breathe normally as you stretch, but emphasize exhaling as you ease deeper into a stretch.
3. Do not force a joint to the point that you feel pain, and do not extend a joint beyond its normal range of motion.
4. Hold each stretch for anywhere from ten to 60 seconds.
5. Ease out of every stretch smoothly and slowly.

To design a stretching program, we recommend you select one stretch for every major muscle group, and for variety, change these stretches at least once a month. To get you started, here are twelve stretches that you can complete in about ten minutes.

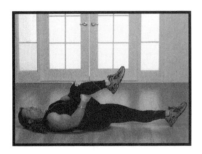

1. Alternate lower back stretch:
Lie prone on a mat or folded towel. Raise one leg up toward your chest. Use your arms to cradle it and increase the stretch. Then repeat for the other leg and alternate for four or five times to loosen the lower back.

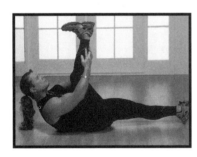

2. Hamstring stretch:
Lie on a mat or folded towel. Raise one leg up as high as possible. Use your arms to pull the leg higher—either from the thigh, calf, or ankle depending on your flexibility. Remember never to stretch to the point where it hurts. Perform for one leg, then alternate with the other for four or five times.

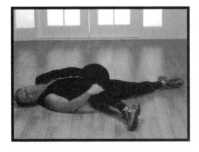

3. Lateral lower back stretch:
Lie on your back on a mat or folded towel and cross your left leg over your right, keeping the left knee bent as shown. Place your right hand on your left leg to hold the stretch. Hold, return, and repeat for the other side.

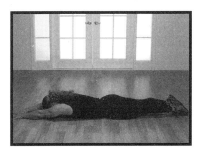

4. Full-Body stretch:

Lie face down on a mat or folded towel and extend your arms in front of you, legs straight behind you. Coming slightly off the floor with arms and legs, stretch to your fullest, pointing your toes. Make yourself as long as possible.

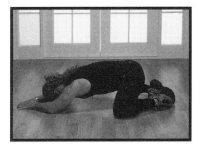

5. Kneeling hip and upper back stretch:

From the position you were just in, come up on your hands and knees. Like a cat, arch your back up and hold, then push your torso down. Repeat several times.

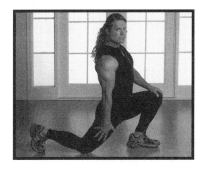

6. Hurdler stretch:

Take a forward stride and bend one knee while letting your trailing foot rest, knee down on the floor behind you. Increase the stretch by pushing forward on the forward knee. Hold and repeat.

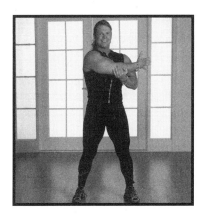

7. Shoulder stretch:

Clasp your elbow with one arm and pull it across the front of your body. Hold, then repeat for the opposite arm. Perform five to six times per arm.

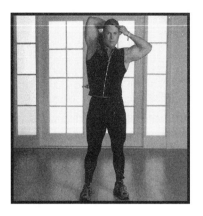

8. Triceps stretch:

Stand with your right arm over your head. Bend your elbow so that your right hand is behind your head. With your left hand, grasp your right wrist and pull back as far as comfortably possible. Hold and repeat with the other arm.

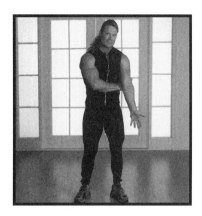

9. Biceps stretch:

Stand with one arm extended, palm up. Place your other hand under your outstretched elbow. Straighten your arm as far as comfortable, pressing the elbow against your other hand. Repeat with the other arm.

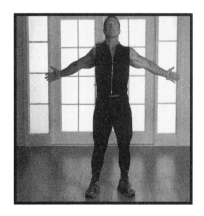

10. Chest stretch:

Stand with your feet shoulder-width apart. Take your arms and stretch them out to the side and toward the back as far as comfortable, then hold. Relax and repeat four or five times.

11. Four-way neck stretch:

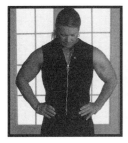 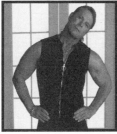 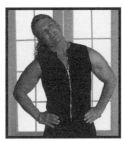 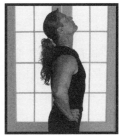

Stand or sit on a chair and gently allow the weight of your head to move forward, right, left, center, and back. You can use your hand for gentle assistance. Be gentle here, don't push it!

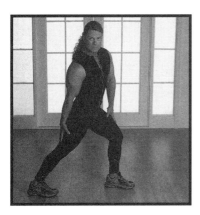

12. Calf muscle stretch:

Stand with your legs as shown. Lower your forward knee to stretch the back of your trailing leg. Perform four or five stretches for one leg before switching to the other.

APPENDIX TWO
Recipes

ON-THE-GO MEALS

▶ Quick Low-Glycemic Chili

4	ounces diced veal, chicken, or beef
½	cup celery, diced
½	green pepper, diced
½	cup mushrooms, sliced
1	cup red kidney beans
2	tablespoons salsa
4	ounces whole canned tomatoes

Mix up and heat in a saucepan for a balanced one-course meal.

▶ Quick South-of-the-Border Burrito

1   reduced-fat tortilla
1   cup chopped vegetables, including broccoli, red peppers, green peppers, onion, and zucchini
2   ounces tofu

Stir-fry the above in 1 teaspoon olive oil in a Pam-sprayed pan. Put into the warmed tortilla. Add 2 tablespoons Mexican cheese and salsa to taste.

Wow! That little bit of salsa is a thermogenic that will help burn the calories you just ate! Whatta deal!

▶ Super-Fast Stir-Fry Chop Suey

1   tablespoon water
4   hearts of baby bok choy
1   cup bean sprouts
½   cup celery, chopped
½   medium bell pepper, chopped
½   cup mushrooms, sliced
¼   cup snow peas
½   cup onion, chopped
5   ounces skinless chicken breast, cut into strips

In a wok or large frying pan coated with Pam, stir-fry the above in 1 tablespoon olive oil.

In last 30 seconds add 2 tablespoons soy sauce and ½ cup steamed slow-cooked rice (white or brown).

SIT-DOWN MEALS

▶ Mediterranean Tomato Salad

Serves 6

6-8	medium Italian plum tomatoes, sliced
8	Kalamata olives, pitted and chopped
1	tablespoon onion, grated
1	tablespoon balsamic vinegar or red wine vinegar
1	tablespoon honey
½	teaspoon salt
¼	teaspoon black pepper, or to taste
½	teaspoon ground cinnamon, or to taste
1	large garlic clove, crushed or minced
1	tablespoon extra-virgin olive oil
2	tablespoons nonfat or low-fat yogurt, preferably plain
	Chopped fresh parsley, for garnish
	Kalamata olives, for garnish (optional)

Arrange the sliced tomatoes and chopped olives attractively on a serving platter. Place onion, vinegar, honey, salt, pepper, cinnamon, and garlic in a jar with a tight-fitting lid. Cover the jar and shake. Don't worry if ingredients don't blend thoroughly. Taste for balance, adding ingredients as desired. Add the oil and shake again.

Drizzle the dressing over the tomato platter and chill for at least 30 minutes.

Just before serving, stir the yogurt and thin with a little water if it won't drizzle off the end of the spoon. Drizzle the yogurt over the tomatoes. Garnish with chopped parsley and more Kalamata olives, if desired.

PER SERVING: Calories 65, Protein 1 g, Carbohydrates 9 g.

▶ Summer Delight Fruit Salad

Serves 12 to 15

1	watermelon
1	cantaloupe
1	honeydew melon
2	cups seedless grapes
	Seasonal fresh fruit (peaches, nectarines, berries, and so on.)
	Lemon juice or apple juice

Slice watermelon in half lengthwise. Remove the fruit from the watermelon using a melon baller. Cut a saw-toothed or scalloped edge on the watermelon shell. Ball or chunk the cantaloupe and honeydew. Mix all the melons and grapes in a large bowl. Dip banana slices in lemon or apple juice to prevent darkening. Add to melons and grapes. Mix carefully. Spoon fruit into the watermelon shell. Cover with plastic wrap and chill 1 to 2 hours.

PER SERVING: Calories 170, Total fat 1.9 g., Protein 3.06 g., Carbohydrates 39.9 g.

▶ Pasta/Veggie Salad

Serves 6

For the salad:

6   ounces spiral noodles

2   cups zucchini squash (¼-inch-thick slices)

2   tomatoes, chopped

½   cup red bell peppers, chopped

½   cup yellow bell peppers, chopped

½   cup green onion, sliced

¼   cup Parmesan cheese

For the dressing:

⅓   cup white wine vinegar

¼   cup seasoned rice vinegar

1   teaspoon olive oil

2   garlic cloves, minced

½   teaspoon dried basil

     Dash salt

¼   teaspoon black pepper

Cook noodles in a large pot of rapidly boiling salted water for 10 to 15 minutes or until tender. While noodles are cooking, prepare the dressing. Combine the vinegars, olive oil, garlic, basil, and salt and pepper. Chill.

Place zucchini in a shallow two-quart casserole. Add 2 tablespoons of water and cover. Microwave for 2½ to 5 minutes. Stir, cover again, and let stand 2 to 3 minutes to finish the cooking process.

Drain pasta and combine with all the vegetables. Pour dressing over the vegetable-pasta mixture and toss. Sprinkle with Parmesan cheese and serve.

> **PER SERVING:** Calories 91.9, Total fat, 2.45 g., Protein 4.35 g., Carbohydrates 14.5 g.

▶ Taco Salad

Serves 6 to 8

½   pound extra-lean ground beef

1   medium onion, chopped (optional if using taco seasoning mix)

1   1¼-ounce package taco seasoning mix or 1 tablespoon chili powder and ½ teaspoon cumin

1   15-ounce can kidney beans or pinto beans, undrained

1   cup cooked brown rice

1   head lettuce, torn into bite-sized pieces

4   medium tomatoes, diced

1   cup low-fat cheese, finely grated (optional)

3–4   cups low-fat corn tortilla chips

      Salsa or mild taco sauce

      Fat-free Ranch or Catalina dressing

Brown the ground beef and onion. Drain off excess fat. Add taco mix or seasoning and beans. Simmer 10 to 15 minutes. Stir in rice and let cool 5 to 10 minutes while you prepare remaining ingredients. Mix lettuce, tomato, and cheese in a large serving bowl. Add meat mixture and slightly crushed chips just before serving. Toss lightly. Serve immediately with salsa and salad dressing.

PER SERVING: Calories 221, Total fat 6.85 g., Protein 16.5 g., Carbohydrates 23.9 g.

▶ Shrimp Supreme

Serves 3

½	pound medium-sized shrimp, cooked and peeled
1	cup seedless red grapes, halved
½	cup celery, sliced on the diagonal
3	ounces water chestnuts, sliced
½	cup golden raisins
8	ounces fresh pineapple, peeled, cored, and diced
1	cup nonfat plain yogurt
1	tablespoon honey
1	tablespoon light teriyaki sauce
1	tablespoon curry powder
	Dash cayenne
2	cups red cabbage, shredded
2	tablespoons fresh parsley, chopped, for garnish

Mix shrimp, grapes, celery, water chestnuts, raisins, and pineapple together in a bowl. Set aside. In a small bowl, mix the yogurt, honey, teriyaki sauce, curry powder, and cayenne. Pour the dressing over the shrimp mixture and blend thoroughly. Arrange the cabbage on the plates and pile the shrimp mixture on top. Garnish with parsley.

PER SERVING: Calories 362, Total Fat 2.86 g., Protein 23 g., Carbohydrates 72 g.

SMOOTHIE RECIPES

▶ Strawberry Banana Smoothie

1   cup frozen strawberries

1   cup of ice

8–10 ounces of Crystal Light (strawberry kiwi, tropical punch), or 4 ounces orange
     juice and 4 ounces water

½   banana

1   scoop (approximately 1 ounce) of egg white protein powder or soya powder

Blend.

▶ Double Chocolate Delight

8   ounces chocolate soy milk (silk) or lowfat milk

1   sugar-free Swiss Miss pack

½   banana

1–2 cups of ice

Blend.

▶ Orange Blast

8   ounces orange juice
1   cup of ice
1   scoop (approximately 1 ounce) of egg white protein powder or soy powder

Blend.

▶ Peachey Queen

1   ripe peach (washed and cut up)
1   cup of ice
1   scoop (approximately 1 ounce) of egg white protein powder or soy powder
6   ounces chocolate soy milk (silk) or lowfat milk
1   teaspoon honey or sugar substitute

Blend.

◢ Sweet Raspberry Delight

2   cups raspberries
2   cups soy milk or lowfat milk
1   cup of ice
1   teaspoon honey or sugar substitute
1   scoop (approximately 1 ounce) of egg white protein powder or soy powder

Blend.

◢ Mango Fandango with Strawberries

2   cups fresh, canned, or frozen mango pieces
12   large strawberries
     Freshly squeezed juice from 1 lemon
1   cup soy milk or lowfat milk

Blend.

TONY LITTLE
Adversity to Victory

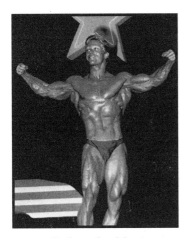
Before Accident

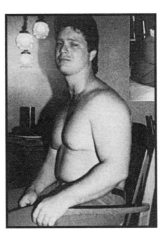
After Accident

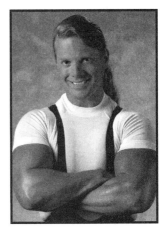
Before Second Accident

TONY LITTLE IS the example of weathering adversity to achieve victory. Tony has succeeded against all odds, and with strong convictions and a deep caring for people, he has brought physical fitness into mainstream America in a way that has enhanced the physical appearance, personal stamina, and emotional outlook of his trainees.

In 1983 Tony was an acclaimed Junior National Bodybuilding Champion, and ready for the big time. He was training for The Mr. America Bodybuilding Championship, the biggest competition of his life, which he was sure he would win.

Then, six months before the competition Tony was blindsided by a school bus. He suffered numerous lacerations to his body and face, two herniated discs, a cracked vertebra, and a dislocated knee. He also experienced massive pain and discomfort throughout his entire body. Though his body had been shattered, he competed in the event and finished in an amazing fifth place. Months following the accident, and the competition, he slowly fell into a depression that resulted in the gradual death of the goals he had set earlier in life. He became hooked on painkillers and nearly 60 pounds overweight. Tony had hit rock bottom.

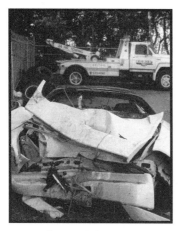
Second Accident

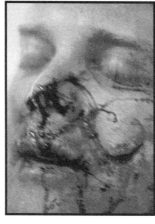
After Second Accident

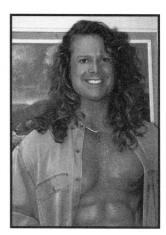
Recovered

One morning in February 1985 Tony felt he had enough of the self-pity and downward spiraling. While he had felt "justified" in wasting his life and blaming his circumstances on his current state, he knew in his heart that the only way to improve his situation was to take control of his life. That began with getting healthy, physically fit, and self-confident. Having spent many days watching various celebrities working out and promoting their gimmicks, diet fads and celebrity fitness videos, he was well-versed on what America was being told about fitness, and he didn't like it. As a certified personal trainer, physical fitness specialist and former national body-building champion, he knew there was much more to getting into shape than aerobic exercise. He also knew that physical strength and mental fortitude was the other part of the equation. So he developed a motivational non-impact resistance exercise technique that would reshape, redesign, and restrengthen the body with minimal joint stress. He knew all too well that poor physical shape is the first *negative* step toward emotional failures and he wanted to be sure that his students were going to feel better and look better in a short period of time by exercising properly.

Tony believed in his idea and was determined to be successful. Armed with faith and confidence in his program, he drummed up his last spark of passion and drive, and went to find out what it would take to make an exercise television show where he could promote his one-on-one approach. A local cable company told him that it would take at least $15,000 to produce a limited local access program, so he started a company cleaning health clubs to raise the necessary capital. His show became a hit. Finally, in 1987, Tony met the president and founder of Home Shopping Network, and they struck a deal. If Tony could sell 400 of his videos in four airings, then they could work together on other projects. It worked; Tony sold all 400 videos in four minutes! His success was due to the fact that he was the first person to spend the majority of the time on his video discussing motivational exercise technique along with muscle group information. Solid, sound advice became his trademark.

This opportunity catapulted his career to new heights. He had proven to himself that he had the knowledge of a personal training style that people were craving. Tony continued his quest to get America back in shape. In a very short time at the Home Shopping Network he broke nearly every one of their records for personal training videos and equipment. People were now starting to know Tony Little, his passion for personal training, and, more important, his *passion for people*. While still working with the Home Shopping Network, Tony decided to try to reach a larger audience by doing infomercials. In 1993 he had record-breaking infomercials in the United States and Europe. Tony then decided to team up with another major shopping network, QVC, and like his time at the Home Shopping Network, it didn't take long for him to start breaking records. Tony's life had become everything he had ever wanted professionally. He had numerous record-breaking sales for his videos and exercise equipment. He had number-one infomercials in several countries and received plenty of awards. And, of course, what got him into all of this in the first place? He was helping people change their bodies and minds worldwide.

Life couldn't have been better for the blond-haired, lean, mean, energized personal training machine. However, in 1996, life threw Tony another curve. He was involved in another life-threatening car accident. His face was severely damaged, especially the left side. He required more than 180 stitches, and this accident took out two more lower back discs, now affecting four out of his five lower back supporting discs. Needless to say, Tony was worried about his well-being and his career. Some people would have thrown in the towel after everything Tony had endured, but he used this obstacle as another way to give himself the motivation to do what God had intended him to do: help people get in shape. In 1998, on New Year's Eve, Tony blasted through the record books. He sold over 200 tractor-trailer truckloads of his Gold Gazelle Glider™ on QVC.

His devotion to helping others combined with his dynamic personality, energy levels beyond reality, and personal before-and-after story have made Tony a favorite among both the public and the media as he continues to capture the attention of audiences worldwide. He has appeared on everything from late night and daytime talk shows such as *The Tonight Show with Jay Leno* and *Ricki Lake* to prominent news broadcasts including CNN and *ABC World News Tonight* among others. Tony has also been featured in such reputable print media as the *Wall Street Journal, USA Today,* the *Los Angeles Times, The New York Times,* as well as hundreds of health, fitness, general interest, and celebrity publications.

Today Tony is still breaking records as he continues to bring the fitness world new ways to get off the couch and get back in shape. His current accolades include thirteen Platinum Video Awards, nine Gold Video Awards, and record-breaking infomercials throughout 81 countries. More than 30 million people worldwide have benefited from his exercise programs. Without a doubt, Tony knows the formula for success. His life has been a painful one at times, but his attitude on overcoming obstacles is simple—Conceive, Believe, and Achieve™.

INDEX

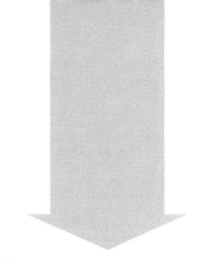

Page numbers in *italic* indicate illustrations; those in **bold** indicate tables.